Improving Aging and Public Health Research

Qualitative and Mixed Methods

Leslie Curry
Renée Shield
Terrie Wetle

Editors

American Public Health Association

Gerontological Society of America
Washington, DC

American Public Health Association
800 I Street, NW
Washington, DC 20001–3710
www.apha.org

Library of Congress Cataloging-in-Publication Data
Improving aging and public health research : qualitative and mixed methods / Leslie
  Curry, Renée Shield, Terrie Welte, editors
        p. cm.
  Includes bibliographical references and index.
  ISBN 0-87553-051-6
        1. Aging--Research. 2. Gerontology--Research. 3. Od age--Research. I. Curry,
  Leslie. II. Shield, Renée Rose. III. Welte, Terrie Todd, 1946-

RA564.8.I47 2006
612.6'7072--dc22   2006049902

Georges C. Benjamin, MD, FACP
Executive Director

Publications Board Liaison: Nancy Persily

Printed and bound in the United States of America
Set In: Book Antiqua and Myriad
Interior Design and Typesetting: Terry Anderson
Cover Design: Irma Rodenhuis
Printing and Binding by Automated Graphic Systems, White Plains, Maryland

ISBN-13: 978-0-87553-051-2
ISBN# 0-87553-051-6

800   10/06

Table of Contents

Foreword   *Charles F. Longino, Jr., PhD*
President, Gerontological Society of America v

Chapter 1   The Unique Contributions of Qualitative and Mixed
Methods to Aging and Public Health Research
Leslie A. Curry, Renée R. Shield, and Terrie Wetle 1

Chapter 2   Qualitative Methods Today
Jaber F. Gubrium 15

Chapter 3   Cultural Forces in the Acceptance of Qualitative Research:
Advancing Mixed Method Research
Mark Luborsky and Andrea Sankar 27

Chapter 4   Qualitative Data Collection for Aging Research:
Choosing the Right Method
Shoshanna Sofaer 39

Chapter 5   "Connected Contributions"as a Motivation for Combining
Qualitative and Quantitative Methods
David L. Morgan 53

Chapter 6   Principles and Procedures of Maintaining Validity
for Mixed-Method Design
Janice M. Morse, Ruth R. Wolfe, and Linda Niehaus 65

Chapter 7   If Not, Why Not? Synchronizing Qualitative and
Quantitative Research in Studying the Elderly
Jay Sokolovsky 79

Chapter 8   Codes to Theory: A Critical Stage in Qualitative Analysis
Elizabeth H. Bradley and Leslie A. Curry 91

Chapter 9   Preserving Cultural Integrity through Analysis
Yewoubdar Beyene 103

Chapter 10   State of the Art: Integrating Software with Qualitative
Analysis
Raymond C. Maietta 117

Chapter 11 Writing a Credible and Fundable Proposal for Qualitative
Research
*Toni Tripp-Reimer, Stacie Salsbury Lyons, Nancy Goldsmith, and
Katherine Bussinger* 141

Chapter 12 Qualitative Research in Gerontology: Preparing a Credible
and Publishable Manuscript
Sara A. Quandt 165

Chapter 13 A Publishable Manuscript: One Editor's Experience and
Recommendations
Linda S. Noelker 175

Chapter 14 Informing Aging-Related Health Policy Through Qualitative
Research
Leslie A. Curry, Renée R. Shield, and Terrie Wetle 183

Index 197

List of Contributors .... .201

Foreword

It is an amazing experience to count the number of papers published in the social sciences section of the *Journals of Gerontology* that are drawn from large data sets, often panel studies, conducted by others. The authors have never looked into the eyes of even one research subject and asked a question. We have become mass consumers of secondary data. The respondents, those in the sample, are faceless abstractions. They seem to have no identities. In this circumstance, we tend to lose sight of the person and instead manipulate categories and levels: health, disability, poverty, marital status, race, and so on. Perhaps that is the nature of most social science research. The strengths and contributions of *both* quantitative and qualitative methodologies, however, are essential to providing insight and solutions to our pressing questions. Although my own research primarily has been based on census data and other large existing data sets, encouraging and legitimating qualitative research in the field of gerontology has been a passion of mine for two decades. As a gerontologist and a professor of public health sciences, I am particularly pleased that this volume addresses how practical applications of qualitative and mixed methods research can be used to illuminate gerontological and public health issues.

At long last, a book has arrived that offers sound advice and insights to researchers wishing to apply qualitative and mixed methods, a book that provides practical tools for designing research, writing grant applications and publishing findings. The importance of these methods is especially timely to address health disparities for work with vulnerable populations.

This book combines theoretical contexts and practical considerations in a refreshingly useful manner. At the same time, it candidly describes the challenges and pitfalls experienced in qualitative and mixed methods research. It teaches how to put a human face on research findings. These approaches are vital to advance the scientific knowledge base in aging and public health. From my work as editor of the *Journal of Gerontology: Social Sciences*, I am particularly pleased to note the fine chapters focusing on writing credible scientific manuscripts and improving the quality of reporting of qualitative research. The practical advice provided by these highly respected scientists will be invaluable to seasoned researchers as well as emerging scientists just setting out on their careers. This much-needed resource should be well used.I am delighted to recommend this text to a diverse audience of readers, from professors to graduate students across a wide range of disciplines. I am certain they will find it valuable as a guide.

Charles F. Longino, Jr., Ph.D., President,
Gerontological Society of America, and
Professor of Sociology and of Public Health Sciences
Wake Forest University

Acknowledgments

This book grows out of two workshops held in conjunction with annual meetings of Gerontological Society of America. In addition to recognizing the expert perspectives on qualitative and mixed methods provided by the presenters and participants, the editors acknowledge support from the John A. Hartford Foundation, the Robert Wood Johnson Foundation, and the National Institute of Aging, NIH (AG024790-01).

Chapter 1

The Unique Contributions of Qualitative and Mixed Methods to Aging and Public Health Research

Leslie Curry, PhD, MPH, Renée Shield, PhD, and Terrie Wetle, MS, PhD

Introduction

This introductory chapter provides a brief overview of the emergence of qualitative and mixed methods approaches in aging and public health research, and highlights the unique and important contributions such methods have made to the scientific literature. We describe the potential role of qualitative approaches in the development of measurement instruments and conceptual models. While recognizing the need for enhanced quality and credibility of qualitative and mixed methods in scientific inquiry, we appeal for greater appreciation of the particular strengths offered by multiple approaches. The chapter closes with an overview of the organization of the volume and a description of each of the chapters.

Applying Qualitative and Mixed Methods in Aging Research

Qualitative methods have been central to research in sociology and anthropology for nearly a century, beginning with the sociological work of the "Chicago school" in the 1920s and the anthropological field studies of Malinowski and others.[1] Since that time, other social and behavioral science disciplines have increasingly employed qualitative approaches. Most recently, qualitative methods have been adopted in health-related research, framing studies in biomedical science,[2] health services research,[3,4] and clinical research.[5-8] Qualitative and mixed methods have been regarded as particularly appropriate for research in aging.[9,10] Such approaches have been applied to the study of end-of-life care;[11-17] health conditions such as Alzheimer's Disease;[18,19] Medicare insurance decisions;[20] health care relationships;[21,22] long term care financing behaviors;[23,24] supportive housing environments such as assisted living;[25] and experiences of professional caregivers in nursing homes.[26-28]

Applying Qualitative and Mixed Methods in Research with Racially and Ethnically Diverse Populations

Significant attention is being directed toward improving our understanding of health, health service use, and health disparities among racially and ethnically diverse older populations. Disentangling the multifactorial causation of health disparities and providing deeper understanding of observed disparities in outcomes may be best accomplished through multi-method approaches. Qualitative studies, including ethnogerontology,[29] which often examines racial, ethnic, and cultural processes of aging qualitatively, have addressed variability and disparities in health in later life,[30] and explored culturally determined values and health beliefs regarding end-of-life care,[31-35] health care treatment seeking behaviors,[36-38] caregiving experiences,[28] and sites of care, such as nursing homes.[39-42]

Focused anthropological attention on aging has used qualitative methodology to probe culturally diverse responses to aging since the seminal work of Clark and Anderson.[43] A range of methods is needed in studying experiences and outcomes among diverse racial and ethnic minority groups, older gay and lesbian populations and immigrants historically underrepresented in research.[44-48] Equally fundamental, by respecting and utilizing native understandings about time, age, and health, qualitative research is ideally suited to reveal, challenge, and confront unexamined assumptions underlying current clinical and scientific practices. This framework is vital to our understanding of an increasingly diverse, complex, and aging population.

Using Qualitative Methods to Inform Evidence-Based Public Health

Qualitative and mixed methods can offer public health research important benefits. In public health, as in medicine, there is emphasis on evidence-based practice.[49] Evidence-based public health practice involves the "use of epidemiological insight while studying and applying research, clinical and public health experience and findings in clinical practice, health programs, and health policies."[50] While the public health empirical literature provides much of the information required for evidence-based public health, crucial gaps remain that limit our ability to develop effective public health policies and to provide optimal public health programs and practices. Strategies for addressing these "evidence gaps" vary, depending upon the issue under study, the content of the current database, and the goals and objectives driving the collection of new knowledge. McKinlay and Marceau[51] argue that we must rethink the most appropriate methodology for public health. This task requires adaptation and refinement of traditional quantitative research methods, such as social surveys and conventional experimental designs, and the inclusion of qualitative methods to complement these more traditional approaches. Whitehead et al.,[52] in examining health inequalities, refer to this as the "evidence jigsaw."

It should also be noted that the factors influencing public health decision making go well beyond the relevant data available. In addition to the scientific soundness of the study and the resultant data, decision makers are affected by how they view the source of the information; the perceived validity of the data; their role and willingness to accept risk and uncertainty; and the environment and context in which the decision is being made, including the culture, timing, media attention, and political constraints.[53] The stage of decision-making also influences the types of data and studies viewed as most appropriate. In their ground-breaking book, *Evidence-Based Public Health*, Brownson and colleagues[49] describe several steps in the process of applying evidence; including assessing scientific evidence; understanding and applying specific analytic tools; developing an initial statement of the issue; quantifying the issue; organizing information from the literature; developing and prioritizing program options; developing and implementing a plan of action; and evaluating the program or policy. At each of these stages, qualitative and mixed methods research may play an important role in contributing to the evidence base.

The step of assessment of the scientific evidence may, for example, involve expert consensus panels or focus groups, while developing the initial statement of the public health issue may use a mixture of qualitative and quantitative strategies. Brownson et al.[49] cite the development of a national influenza vaccination program for elders as an example. Quantitative survey data can provide estimates of vaccination rates among older adults, while qualitative data describe potential barriers older adults face in receiving vaccinations. Together, these methods suggest potential strategies to boost vaccination rates. Efforts to quantify the public health problem frequently benefit from mixed methods strategies, and are useful in assuring that the quantitative data are both valid and relevant. Developing and prioritizing program options rely on evidence to determine types of options that are most acceptable to target populations, program designs that are culturally appropriate, and implementation strategies that are effective and well received by intended participants. The process of creating the action plan and implementing interventions is also enhanced by qualitative strategies, especially those that involve key stakeholders, including the intervention's target audiences. For example, focus groups help identify preferred strategies and barriers to implementation, and also can help to achieve programmatic "buy-in." The final stage described by Brownson et al.[49] is the evaluation of the program or public health policy. Evaluation data include a wide range of measures, the most effective of which include qualitative information derived from interviews, diaries, content analyses of press materials, observations, or focus groups. These sorts of data provide the rich texture of response to the program and provide deeper understanding of the more quantitative outcome data collected in most evaluations.

Using Qualitative Research to Develop Quantitative Measures

In addition to the specific contributions of qualitative and mixed methods to aging and public health research, such approaches can also be used to improve quantitative methodology. For example, various qualitative methods are becoming commonly recognized for their value in informing quantitative measurement processes and instruments. Focus groups, in-depth interviews, cognitive interviews, and participant observation have been employed to develop patient-centered measures of key outcome variables, such as religion in late life,[54] quality of life for individuals with prostate cancer,[55] and other terminal illnesses.[34] Qualitative designs have also been used to construct comprehensive taxonomies that identify core elements of a particular phenomenon as a useful precursor to developing quantitative measures.[56-58] For example, one study employed focus groups to characterize psychosocial considerations in individual decisions to finance long-term care in order to inform subsequent quantitative investigations.[23] Psychological principles and measures that have not been cross-validated with different populations may be based on erroneous assumptions or rely on constructs unfamiliar to the population of interest.[44] Qualitative, exploratory approaches that allow participants to identify concepts of importance and to express them in language that has meaning for that group can provide critical insights into developing culturally literate and relevant measures.[59,60]

Using Qualitative Methods for Building Conceptual Models

In addition to applying qualitative methods to investigate empirical questions, such approaches can guide the development and refinement of conceptual models and theoretical frameworks. Grounded theory, or the discovery of theory from data systematically obtained from social research, has been proposed as an essential first step in the exploration of phenomena that have not been well studied or are poorly understood.[61] This process of hypothesizing inductively from data uses study participants' own concepts to build theoretical frameworks that explain the collected data.[62] For example, a qualitative investigation of a prevailing model of health service use (the Andersen model) suggested modifications that may enhance the model's explanatory power when applied to empirical studies of ethnicity and long term care use.[63] Another example is provided by a qualitative fieldwork study that was used to construct a model of aging-in-place for older adults using adult day care or assisted living services.[64]

Synthesizing Qualitative and Quantitative Methods

Although qualitative and quantitative methods have historically been viewed as mutually exclusive sciences, such rigid distinctions among various modes of scientific inquiry are increasingly recognized as inappropriate and counterproductive. In recent years, qualitative methods have more usefully been seen as both valuable in their own right and as an important complement to quantitative investigations. The concept of "methodological pluralism," or research that draws upon the strengths of both quantitative and qualitative approaches, is becoming accepted and encouraged within a variety of scientific disciplines.[65] Some experts argue that the current question is not whether such methods should be combined, but rather how to best achieve sound methodological and analytic integration. The selection and application of methods must be approached with care, with respectful regard for the analytic traditions from which they spring, and with consideration of how well they are suited for the problem or question at hand. Proponents of mixed methods espouse the value of this multifaceted approach for studying a wide array of issues including clinical conditions such as dementia,[66] health services research such as patterns of service use[67] and health care treatment decisions,[68,69] and studies of ageism in health care.[66] Combining quantitative and qualitative strategies has even been advocated in population and demographic studies.[70]

Need for Improved Quality and Credibility

Despite the steady integration of qualitative methods in health and health services research, concerns about scientific rigor persist, and the dissemination and wide adoption for appropriate research questions remain constrained. Qualitative methods have been criticized for being subject to researcher bias, lacking reproducibility and generalizability, and producing knowledge that is less valuable than that from quantitative sciences.[71] Although there is a lack of widespread consensus on standards of scientific rigor,[72] various guidelines for assessing soundness of qualitative studies have been proposed.[73-76] Particularly challenging is the fact that the standards governing qualitative inquiry vary among qualitative traditions and methods.[74] Nevertheless, there is general agreement that credibility may be enhanced by the use of such procedures as triangulation (gathering a range of data from multiple sources), peer debriefing, transparent reporting of the methods used, external audits, thick description, and searching for confirming and disconfirming cases. The extent to which these strategies are employed and/or presented clearly in research reports is highly variable and generally needs improvement.

The gerontology, geriatrics, and public health literature using qualitative methods is growing, yet journal editors and reviewers caution that the quality of submitted manuscripts remains mixed. Challenges to the effective communication of qualitative research to diverse lay and professional audiences, scientists with a strong orientation to quantitative methods, journal editors, funding agencies, policymakers, and health care providers remain. Frequently due to space limitations, authors of qualitative or mixed method studies cannot provide appropriate detail regarding study design and data analysis in manuscripts.[77] In addition, the peer review of qualitative and mixed methods manuscripts is constrained by the limited guidance for reviewing journal submissions.[78] One recent analysis of funding decisions suggests that qualitative studies frequently receive lower review scores than quantitative studies, in part due to the fact that the qualitative proposals do not provide sufficient detail regarding design and analysis and do not explicitly link methodological strategies to research goals.[79] While the potential of qualitative research for significant contributions to policymaking has been noted, the link between qualitative researchers and the policy community is tenuous at best.[80] Publication of qualitative findings has not been tailored to reach the media, governmental agencies, policymakers, and the lay public.[81] Finally, potential beneficiaries of knowledge gained through qualitative studies, such as health care providers, are not well trained to read critically and identify sound research.[82,83]

Overview of the Book

This edited volume is designed to address many of the barriers to producing and disseminating excellent qualitative and mixed methods research. Intended for scholars with expertise in aging, public health, and related areas, such as health disparities and ethnogerontology; graduate students in varied fields; funding agencies and foundations that support such research; and editors and reviewers from aging-related scientific journals, the volume reviews the critical aspects of conducting methodologically sound and scientifically important inquiry. Written by a group of internationally recognized scientists from a range of disciplines and fields of research with extensive experience in qualitative and mixed methods, the book offers a wide assortment of examples of their work and those of their colleagues. The book addresses theoretical and practical considerations and is organized to generally mirror the research process. The chapters begin with an exploration of the value and need for qualitative methods, and then progress through the tasks and strategies involved in pursuing a research question from generating the idea, conducting the research, and analyzing data. The concluding section presents guidance on preparing grant proposals and disseminating research findings. Each of the chapters is described briefly below.

In the book's "Qualitative Methods in Perspective" section, Chapter 2, Jaber Gubrium, presents the perspective of a highly experienced researcher who began conducting qualitative research in the 1970s. He offers important observations about how the field has evolved in terms of procedural sophistication as well as an increased awareness of the researcher's critical role in shaping the study and its findings. Dr. Gubrium notes that the researcher brings his or her unique methodological and theoretical orientation to each study, which must be explicitly acknowledged. Chapter 3, by Mark Luborsky and Andrea Sankar, explores the question of why qualitative methods have had mixed success in being accepted by mainstream gerontology and public health despite substantial and acknowledged contributions to the literature. Their provocative essay notes the valued place that qualitative methods enjoy in physical sciences, as compared with social sciences and offers examples of this acceptance. Drs. Luborsky and Sankar suggest cultural reasons underlying this familiar reception and challenge the qualitative researcher to improve the scientific rigor and credibility of methods in qualitative inquiry.

The book's second section, "Considerations in Conceptualization and Design," turns to the theoretical and practical aspects of conceiving and conducting sound qualitative and mixed methods studies. Chapter 4, by Shoshanna Sofaer, provides guidance regarding how to determine whether a particular method is appropriate for addressing a specific research question. After reviewing the major qualitative data collection techniques, Dr. Sofaer describes how the data collection method influences data quality, and proposes a methodological research agenda to begin to address the implications of specific data collection choices. In Chapter 5, David Morgan addresses various strategies for combining qualitative and quantitative methods. He notes the importance of examining one's motivation for using mixed methods, and argues that a clear rationale for a given design is essential from the outset. Dr. Morgan then presents a series of mixed methods designs that are defined by sequential priorities of the research. Considerations in mixed methods studies are further explored in Chapter 6 by Janice Morse and others. Focusing on threats to validity inherent in such approaches, They stress that researchers should have a well-conceived plan and justification for including each component. They then define three principles to assist with maintaining the validity of a study. The approaches described in Chapters 5 and 6 are then illustrated by a discussion of a specific body of research. In Chapter 7, Jay Sokolovsky explores the important potential for qualitative and mixed methods in addressing a critical aspect of health—social networks. The study of social networks provides ways to understand how health information and interpersonal support operate in practice. Dr. Sokolovsky is concerned with how qualitative and quantitative methods can work together so that culturally accurate data for specific groups can be reliably compared and generalized. In trying to understand, for example, how a group of urban elderly interact with and rely on one another, he describes an "ethnometric" social network approach for developing culturally appropriate "Network Profiles" that define social linkages and their meaning to informants.

The third section of the book, "Planning and Implementing Scientifically Sound Analyses," brings the reader to the step of data analysis. In Chapter 8, Elizabeth Bradley and Leslie Curry provide a brief overview of fundamental principles and steps in qualitative data analysis and discuss the process of developing coding schemes and coding data. They conclude with a description of how to move from coding to generating research output, including taxonomies of complex phenomena, themes or hypotheses, and conceptual frameworks. The importance of attention to cultural relevance during data analysis is addressed by Yewoubdar Beyene in Chapter 9. Dr. Beyene reviews the strengths of anthropology in examining biological, cultural, ecological, linguistic, and historical factors related to health and illness. Dr. Beyene describes how she has used a variety of methods, including interviews, census taking, and extensive participant observation, in her anthropological research in Mexico, Greece, and Cameroon to explore differences and similarities in perceptions and practices about health behaviors and aging. Noting, for example, that menopausal symptoms in these different societies vary and are not completely explained by role changes and cultural taboos, she demonstrates how culture and biology are complexly involved in this description of her extensive research. This section of the book ends with a chapter to illustrate practical application of these principles of data analysis. In Chapter 10, Ray Maeitta begins by suggesting that software can best be used as an electronic organizer and reliable, dynamic access tool that encourages the researcher to think more creatively and responsibly. He goes on to describe the "Sort and Sift" technique, which encourages frequent movement between thorough review of data and reflections on content and process used during data analysis. This chapter is intended to be highly practical and to give the reader a clear sense of current software capabilities.

The book's final section, "Effectively Communicating Qualitative and Mixed Methods Research," addresses the vital role of writing in all phases of a research endeavor, from the proposal stage to disseminating findings to various audiences, including funding agencies, journal editors, policymakers, and other researchers. These chapters offer practical advice to guide the investigator in these important tasks. In Chapter 11, Toni Tripp-Reimer and her co-authors provide a detailed description of strategies for writing a credible and fundable proposal. The following two chapters address how to prepare a publishable manuscript from the perspectives of a qualitative researcher and a scientific journal editor, respectively. In Chapter 12, Sara Quandt presents a step-by-step review of the challenges and essential steps in writing a credible and compelling research manuscript. She notes the importance of carefully choosing an appropriate target journal, offers guidance for crafting the manuscript, and describes the peer-review process. In Chapter 13, Linda Noelker, editor of *The Gerontologist*, offers her insights as a peer-reviewed scientific journal editor. She begins by an analysis of the volume and publication rate of manuscripts using qualitative and mixed methods. She then reviews in detail the major reasons for rejection of qualitative research submissions and offers a series of specific recommendations to prospective authors. The section then turns to the issue of effectively communicating qualitative research to policymakers. In Chapter 14, Leslie Curry, Renée Shield, and Terrie Wetle begin by describing the potential contributions of qualitative and mixed methods to aging-related policy development. After identifying barriers to effective research dissemination, they discuss approaches to enhancing policymakers' confidence in qualitative research and examine strategies for building essential relationships between the research and aging health policy communities. The chapter closes with a review of specific communication techniques that can enhance the effectiveness of disseminating research findings to policymakers.

It is with much pleasure that this collection of integrated and thoughtful articles is offered to investigators interested in enhancing their research in aging and public health. The theoretical considerations and practical approaches assembled here are offered as a positive way to successfully incorporate qualitative methods into research. Attention to the vital areas described herein promises to reward the reader by demonstrating ways to enhance his/her own research. It is hoped that researchers will be inspired to utilize these contributions in their work, which will proceed to yield important and socially valuable insight into the diverse ways illness, health, and aging are experienced in the world today.

References

1) Denzin, N. and Lincoln, Y. The Discipline and Practice of Qualitative Research. In Denzin, N. and Lincoln, Y. (Eds.). *Handbook of Qualitative Research, 2nd Edition.* 2000; pp.1-28. Thousand Oaks, CA: Sage Ltd.

2) Kaplan, G. and Baron-Epel, O. What Lies Behind the Subjective Evaluation of Health Status? *Social Science and Medicine.* 2003; 56(8):1669-76.

3) Pope, C. and Mays, N. Qualitative Research: Reaching the Parts Other Methods Cannot Reach: An Introduction to Qualitative Methods in Health and Health Services Research. *British Medical Journal.* 1995; 311(6996):42-45.

4) Shortell, S. The Emergence of Qualitative Methods in Health Services Research. *Health Services Research.* 1999; 34(5):1083-1090.

5) Berkwits, M. and Inui, T. Making Use of Qualitative Research Techniques. *Journal of General Internal Medicine.* 1998; 13(3):195-99.

6) Green, J. and Britten, N. Qualitative Research and Evidence Based Medicine. *British Medical Journal.* 1998; 316 (7139):1230-32.

7) Miller, W. and Crabtree, B. Clinical Research. In N.K. Denzin and Y.S. Lincoln (eds.) *Strategies of Qualitative Inquiry, 2nd Edition.* 2003, pp. 397-434. Thousand Oaks, CA: Sage.

8) Schoenberg, N., Amey, C., Stoller, E., and Muldoon, S. Lay Referral Patterns Involved in Cardiac Treatment Decision Making Among Middle-Aged and Older Adults. *The Gerontologist.* 2003 Aug; 43(4):493-502.

9) Cobb, A.K. and Forbes, S. Qualitative Research: What Does it Have to Offer to the Gerontologist? *Journals of Gerontology: Medical Sciences.* 2002; 57A (4):197-202.

10) Gubrium, J. Qualitative Research Comes of Age in Gerontology. *The Gerontologist.* 1992; 32(5):581-2.

11) Back, A., et al. Clinician-Patient Interactions About Requests for Physician-Assisted Suicide: A Patient and Family View. *Archives of Internal Medicine.* 2002; 162(11):1257-65.

12) Curry, L., Schwartz, H., Gruman, C., and Blank, K. Physician's Voices on Physician Assisted Suicide: Looking Beyond the Numbers. *Ethics and Behavior.* 2000; 10(4):337-361

13) Singer, P., Martin, D., and Kelner, M. Quality End-of-Life Care: Patients' Perspectives. *Journal of the American Medical Association.* 1999; 281(2):163-8.

14) Travis, S., Bernard, M., Dixon, S., McAuley, W., Loving, G., and McClanahan, L. Obstacles to Palliation and End-Of-Life Care in a Long-Term Care Facility. *The Gerontologist.* 2002, 42, 3, June, 342-349.

15) Wetle, T., Teno, J., Shield, R., Welch, L., and Miller, S.C. *End of Life in Nursing Homes: Experiences and Policy Recommendations.* 2004. Washington, DC: AARP Public Policy Institute.

16) Shield, R., Wetle, T., Teno, J., Miller, S.C., and Welch, L. Physicians "Missing in Action:" Family Perspectives on Physician and Staffing Problems in End-of-Life Care in the Nursing Home. *J. of the Amer. Geriatr. Soc.* 2005; 53:1651-1657.

17) Wetle, T., Shield, R., Teno, T., Miller, S.C., and Welch, L. Family Perspectives on End-of-Life Care Experiences in Nursing Homes. *The Gerontologist.* 2005; 45 (5): 642-650.

18) Mahoney, D. Vigilance: Evolution and Definition for Caregivers of Family Members with Alzheimer's Disease. *Journal of Gerontological Nursing.* 2003; 29(8):24-30

19) Sanders, S. and Corely, C. Are They Grieving: A Qualitative Analysis Examining Grief in Caregivers of Individuals with Alzheimer's Disease. *Social Work Health Care.* 2003; 37(3):35-53.

20) Sofaer, S., Kreling, B., Kenney, E., Swift, E., and Dewart, T. Family Members and Friends who Help Beneficiaries Make Health Decisions. *Health Care Financing Review.* 2001; 23(1):105-122.

21) Adler, S. Relationships Among Older Patients, CAM Practitioners, and Physicians: The Advantages of Qualitative Inquiry. *Alternative Therapies Health Medicine.* 2003; 9(1):104-110.

22) Gallagher, T., Waterman, A., Ebers, A., Fraser, V., and Levinson, W. Patients' and Physicians' Attitudes Toward the Disclosure of Medical Errors. *JAMA.* 2003; 289(8):1001-7.

23) Curry, L., Bradley, E., and Robison, J. Individual Decisions Regarding Financing Nursing Home Care: Psychosocial Considerations. *Journal of Aging Studies.* 2004; 18(3):337-352.

24) Peters, C. and Pinkston, E. Controllers and Noncontrollers: A Typology of Older Americans and Their Caregivers' Approaches to Managing the Private Funding of Long Term Care. *Qualitative Health Research.* 2002; 12(9):1161-83.

25) Ball, M., Perkins, M., Whittington, F., Connell, B., Hollingsworth, C., King, S., Elrod, C., Combs, B. Managing Decline in Assisted Living: The Key to Aging In Place. *Journals of Gerontology B: Psychological Sciences and Social Sciences.* 2004 Jul; 59(4):S202-12.

26) Diamond, T. *Making Gray Gold: Narratives of Nursing Home Care.* 1992; Chicago: University of Chicago Press.

27) Jervis, L. The Pollution of Incontinence and the Dirty Work of Caregiving in a U.S. Nursing Home. *Medical Anthropology Quarterly.* 2001; 15 (1): 58-83.

28) Foner, Nancy. *The Caregiving Dilemma: Work in an American Nursing Home.* 1994. Berkeley: University of California Press.

29) Applewhite, S. Qualitative Research in Educational Gerontology. *Educational Gerontology.* 1997; 23(1):15-28.

30) Allen, K., Blieszner, R., Roberto, K. Families in Middle and Later Years: A Review and Critique of Research in the 1990s. *Journal of Marriage and Family.* 2000; 62(4):911-927.

31) Hauser, J., Kleefield, S., Brennan, T., Fuschbach, R. Minority Populations and Advance Directives: Insights From Focus Group Methodology. *Cambridge Quarterly of Healthcare Ethics.* 1997; 6(1):58-71

32) Morrison, R.S., Zayas, L.H., Mulvihill, M., Baskin, S.A., and Meier, D.E. Barriers to Completion of Health Care Proxy Forms: A Qualitative Analysis of Ethnic Differences. *Journal of Clinical Ethics.* 1998; 9(2):118-126.

33) Morrow, E. Attitudes of Women from Vulnerable Populations Toward Physician-Assisted Death: A Qualitative Approach. *Journal of Clinical Ethics.* 1997; 8(3):279-89.

34) Tong, E., McGraw, S.A., Dobihal, E., Baggish, R., Cherlin, E., and Bradley, E.H. What is a Good Death? Minority and Non-Minority Views. *Journal of Palliative Care.* 2003; 19:168-175

35) Waters, C. Understanding and Supporting African Americans' Perspectives on End-of-Life Care Planning and Decision Making. *Qualitative Health Research.* 2001; 11(3):385-98.

36) Bates, M., Rankin-Hill, L., and Sanchez-Ayandez, M. The Effects of the Cultural Context of Health Care on Treatment and Response to Chronic Pain and Illness. *Social Science and Medicine.* 1997; 45(9):1433-47.

37) Esser-Stuart, J. and Lyons, M. Barriers and Influences in Seeking Health Care Among Lower Income Minority Women. *Social Work Health Care*. 2002; 35(3):85-99.

38) O'Malley, A., Renteria-Weitzman, R., Huerta, E., and Mandelblatt, J., Latin American Cancer Research Coalition, Patient Provider Priorities for Cancer Prevention and Control: A Qualitative Study in Mid-Atlantic Latinos. *Ethnicity and Disease*. 2002; 12(3):383-391.

39) Janevic, M. and Connell, C. Racial, Ethnic, and Cultural Differences in the Dementia Caregiving Experience: Recent Findings. *The Gerontologist*. 2001; 41(3):334-337.

40) Shield, R. Wary Partners: Family-CNA Relationships in Nursing Homes. In: Stafford, P. (ed.) *Gray Areas: Ethnographic Encounters with Nursing Home Culture*. 2003; Santa Fe: SAR Press.

41) Gubrium, J. *Living and Dying at Murray Manor*. 1975; New York: St. Martin's Press.

42) Shield, R. *Uneasy Endings: Daily Life in an American Nursing Home*. 1988; Ithaca: Cornell University Press.

43) Clark, M. and Anderson, B. *Culture and Aging: An Anthropological Study of Older Americans*. 1967; Springfield: Charles C. Thomas.

44) Weitzman, P. and Levkoff, S. Combining Qualitative and Quantitative Methods in Health Research with Minority Elders: Lessons from a Study of Dementia Caregiving. *Field Methods*. 2000; 12, 3, Aug, 195-208

45) Stewart, A.L. and Napoles-Springer, A. Health-Related Quality-of-Life Assessments in Diverse Population Groups in the United States. *Medical Care*. 2000 Sep; 38(9 Suppl):II102-24.

46) Hash, K. and Cramer, E. Empowering Gay and Lesbian Caregivers and Uncovering their Unique Experiences Through the Use of Qualitative Methods. *Journal of Gay and Lesbian Social Services*. 2003; 15, 1-2, 47-63.

47) Usita, P. and Blieszner, R. Immigrant Family Strengths: Meeting Communication Challenges *Journal of Family Issues*. 2002; 23, 2, Mar, 266-286

48) Weitzman, P.F., Chang, G., Reynoso, H. Middle-Aged and Older Latino American Women in the Patient-Doctor Interaction. *Journal of Cross Cultural Gerontology*. 2004 Sep; 19(3):221-39.

49) Brownson, R.C., Baker, E.A., Leet, T.L., and Gillespie, K.N. *Evidence-Based Public Health*. 2003. New York: Oxford Press.

50) Jenicek, M. Epidemiology, Evidence-Based Medicine, and Evidence-Based Public Health. *Journal of Epidemiology*. 1997; 7: 187-197.

51) McKinlay, J.B. and Marceau, L.D. To Boldly Go.... *American Journal of Public Health*. 2000; 90: 25-33.

52) Whitehead., M., Petticrew, M., Graham, H., MacInntyre, S.J., Bambra, C., and Egan, M. Evidence for Public Health Policy on Inequalities: 2: Assembling the Evidence Jigsaw. *Journal of Epidemiology Community Health*. 2004; 58: 817-821.

53) Bero, L.A., Jahad, A.R. How Consumers and Policy Makers can use Systematic Reviews for Decision Making. In: Mulrow, C. and Cook, D., (eds.) *Systematic Reviews. Synthesis of Best Evidence for Health Care Decisions*. 1998; Philadelphia: American College of Physicians.

54) Krause, N. A Comprehensive Strategy for Developing Closed-Ended Survey Items for Use in Studies of Older Adults. *Journals of Gerontology:Psychological Sciences and Social Sciences*. 2002; 57: S263-S274.

55) Clark, J., Bokhour, B., Inui, T., Silliman, R., and Talcott, J. Measuring Patients' Perceptions of the Outcomes of Treatment for Early Prostate Cancer. *Medical Care*. 2003; 41(8):923-36.

56) Bradley, E.H., Holmboe, E., Mattera, J., Roumani, S., Radford, M.J., and Krumholz, H.K. A Qualitative Study of Increasing Beta-Blocker Use After Myocardial Infarction: Why do Some Hospitals Succeed? *JAMA*, .2001; 285:2604-2611.

57) Prigerson, H., Cherlin, E., Chen, J., Kasl, S.V., Johnson-Hurzeler, R., and Bradley, E.H. The Stressful Caregiving Adult Reactions to Experiences of Dying (SCARED) Scale: Measure to Assess Caregiver Exposures and Responses in Terminal care. *American Journal of Geriatric Psychiatry*. 2003; 11:309-319.

58) Studenski, S. Hayes, R.P., Leibowitz, R.Q., Bode, R., Lavery, L., Walston, J., Duncan, P. and Perera S. Clinical Global Impression of Change in Physical Frailty: Development of a Measure Based on Clinical Judgment. *Journal of the American Geriatrics Society*. 2004 Sep; 52(9):1560-6.

59) Carter-Edwards, L., Bynoe, M., and Svetkey, L. Knowledge of Diet and Blood Pressure Among African Americans: Use of Focus Groups for Questionnaire Development. *Ethnicity and Disease*.1998; 8:184-97.

60) Gubrium, J., Rittman, M., Williams, C., Young, M., and Boylstein, C. Benchmarking as Everyday Functional Assessment in Stroke Recovery. *Journals of Gerontology B: Psychological and Social Sciences*. 2003; 58(4):S203-211.

61) Glaser, B. and Strauss, A. *The Discovery of Grounded Theory: Strategies for Qualitative Research*. 1967; Chicago: Aldine.

62) Charmaz, K. Grounded Theory: Objectivist and Constructivist Methods. In Denzin, N. and Lincoln, Y. (eds.). *Strategies of Qualitative Inquiry, 2nd edition*, pp. 249-291. 2003; Thousand Oaks, CA: Sage Ltd.

63) Bradley, E., McGraw, S., Curry, L., Buckser, A., King, K., Kasl, S., and Andersen, R. Expanding the Andersen Model: The Role of Psychosocial Factors in Long-Term Care Use. *Health Services Research*. 2002; 37(5):1221-1242

64) Cutchin, M. The Process of Mediated Aging-in-Place: A Theoretically and Empirically Based Model. *Social Science Medicine*. 2003; 57 (6):1077-90.

65) Morse, J.M. Qualitative Methods: The State of the Art. *Qualitative Health Research*. 1999; 9(3):393-406.

66) Bond, J. and Corner, L. Researching Dementia: Are There Unique Methodological Challenges for Health Services Research? *Aging and Health*. 2001; 21(1):95.

67) Vig, E., Devenport, N., and Pearlman, R. Good Deaths, Bad Deaths and Preferences for the End of Life: A Qualitative Study of Geriatric Outpatients. *Journal of the American Geriatrics Society*. 2002; 50(9):1541-49.

68) Jenkins, C. Care Arrangement Decisions for Frail Older Women: Quantitative and Qualitative Perspectives. *Journal of Women and Aging*. 2000; 12, 3-4, 3-20.

69) Tsuchiya, A., Dloan, P., and Shaw, R. Measuring People's Preferences Regarding Ageism in Health: Some Methodological Issues and Some Fresh Evidence. *Social Science Medicine*. 2003; 54(7):687-96.

70) Knodel, J. A Case for Nonanthropological Qualitative Methods for Demographers. *Population and Development Review*. 1997; 23(4):847-54.

71) Mays, N. and Pope, C. Assessing Quality in Qualitative Research. *British Medical Journal*. 2000; 320:50-52.

72) Devers, K. How will we Know "Good" Qualitative Research When We See It? *Health Services Research* . 1999; 24(5): 1153-1188.

73) Creswell, J. *Qualitative Inquiry and Research Design: Choosing Among Five Traditions*. 1998; Thousand Oaks: Sage Ltd.

74) Frankel, R. Standards of Qualitative Research. In Crabtree, B. and Miller, W. (eds.). *Doing Qualitative Research, 2nd Edition* (pp. 333-347). 1999; Newbury Park, CA:Sage.

75) Patton, M. Enhancing the Quality and Credibility of Qualitative Analysis. *Health Services Research.* 1999; 34(5): 1189-1208.

76) Smith, J. and Deemer, D. The Problem of Criteria in an Age of Relativism. In: Denzin, D.K. and Lincoln, Y.S. (Eds.) *Handbook of Qualitative Research, 2nd Edition,* 2000; Thousand Oaks, CA: Sage

77) Mays, N. and Pope, C. Qualitative Research: Rigor and Qualitative Research. *British Medical Journal.* 1995; 311(6997):109-112.

78) Popay, J. Rogers, A., and Williams, G. Rationale and Standards for the Systematic Review of Qualitative Literature in Health Services Research. *Qualitative Health Research.* 1998; 8(3):341-351.

79) Belgrave, L., Zablotsky, D., and Guadagno, M. How do We Talk to Each Other? Writing Qualitative Research For Quantitative Readers. *Qualitative Health Research.* 2002; 12(10):1427-39.

80) Rist, R. Influencing the Policy Process with Qualitative Research. In Denzin N and Lincoln Y (Eds.) *Handbook of Qualitative Research, 2nd Edition,* 2000; pp:1001-1017.Thousand Oaks, CA: Sage Publications

81) Kayser-Jones, J. Malnutrition, Dehydration, and Starvation in the Midst of Plenty: The Political Impact of Qualitative Inquiry. *Qualitative Health Research.* 2002; 12(10):1391-405.

82) Giacomini, M. and Cook, D. Users' Guides to the Medical Literature: XXIII. Qualitative Research in Health Care A. Are the Results of the Study Valid? Evidence-Based Medicine Working Group. *Journal of the American Medical Association.* 2000; 284(3):357-62.

83) Giacomini, M. and Cook, D. Users' Guides to the Medical Literature:XXIII. Qualitative Research in Health Care B. What are the Results and How do They Help me Care for my Patients? *Journal of the American Medical Association.* 2000; 284(3):357-62.

Additional Resources

Allison, R.A. and Foster, J.E. Measuring Health Equality Using Qualitative Data. *Journal of Health Economics.* 2004; 23:505-524.

Harden, A., Garcia, J., Oliver, S., Rees, R., Shepherd, J., Brunton, G., and Oakley, A. Applying Systematic Review Methods to Studies of People's Views: An Example From Public Health Research. *Journal of Epidemiology Community Health.* 2004; 58: 794-800.

O'Neall, M.A. and Brownson, R.C. Teaching Evidence-Based Public Health to Public Health Practitioners, 2004; *Annals of Epidemiology.*

Pettigrew, M., Whitehead, M., Macintyre, S.J., Graham, H., and Egan, M. Evidence for Public Health Policy on Inequalities: 1: The Reality According to Policymakers. *Journal of Epidemiology Community Health.* 2004; 58: 811-816.

Chapter 2

Qualitative Methods Today

Jaber F. Gubrium, PhD

Introduction

I am pleased to comment on qualitative methods today on the occasion of the publication of this important volume on qualitative and mixed methods in aging and public health research. It is important for two reasons. One is that skilled and experienced qualitative researchers bring to bear the latest methodological and analytic considerations on an orientation to the empirical world that has gained enormous respect and widespread acceptance in the last two decades. The second reason is that their considerations refer to a substantive area—aging, public health concerns, and health disparities—that is looming in importance as populations rapidly grow older and their well-being becomes a significant social issue. The combination is a mark of distinction as qualitative researchers in aging engage their craft.

Increased Reflexivity of the Research Role

Qualitative methods today are not the same as when they first appeared on the procedural horizon. Whether the methods refer to in-depth interviews, participant observation, the analysis of textual and visual material, or a combination of these, what is being done now is more reflexive than ever. Simply put, the qualitative researcher now recognizes that the research role requires examination. The qualitative researcher must be self-aware and include him or herself in the examination. Qualitative researchers now have a greater sense that what is done under the aegis of procedure at least in part constructs the empirical contours of the subject matter under consideration.[1] Data on the one hand, and methods and analysis on the other, are no longer viewed as separate and distinct. What data are and how the empirical world is viewed in the first place draw significantly from the orienting framework that researchers put into place as they do their work. It has become increasingly clear in these decades that what the researcher selects to study and chooses to observe, count, and describe derive from a theoretical perspective that the researcher must acknowledge explicitly. The recognition that methodology and theoretical stance are not neutral and provide a determining lens on the research has had momentous effect.

The Historical Context of Qualitative Methods

A historical comparison is instructive. In the 1840s, British social researcher Henry Mayhew[2] touted the urgency of moving beyond "government population returns" in investigating the then-unknown lives of London's "humbler classes." Knowledge was to be drawn from "the lips of the people themselves—giving a literal description of their labor, their earnings, their trials, and their sufferings, in their own 'unvarnished' language" (p. xv). Anthropologists applied this orientation to the comparative study of cultures worldwide. In the American context, W. I. Thomas and Florian Znaniecki's[3] monumental study of the immigration experience of Poles to Chicago, published in 1918, claimed empirical perfection in the experiential details of the series of letters they collected from Polish families in Chicago and in Poland. As the authors write at the end of volume two, "We are safe in saying that personal life-records, as complete as possible, constitute the perfect type of sociological material . . . ." (p. 1832). In other words, it was suggested that what people said and how they said it might be considered a different, and perhaps superior, report than what others said about them.

Decades later, at mid-century, William Foote Whyte[4] repeats the call for a method of procedure that can secure a similar sense of unvarnished data, hailing the value of intensive participant observation. Referring to statistical information about Cornerville, an Italian slum in Eastern City, Whyte prods the reader when he compares the thin lives portrayed by available statistics with the results of careful fieldwork: "In this [statistical] view, Cornerville people appear as social work clients, as defendants in criminal cases, or as undifferentiated members of 'the masses.' There is one thing wrong with this picture: no human beings are in it" (p. xv). As if to say that human beings come alive by way of a qualitative method of procedure, Whyte then presents the intricate social structure of an Italian slum.

Relevance for Gerontology

Applied to older people and the aging experience, the procedural sentiments of these early years are evident. It is considered worthy to capture the experiences and perspectives of older people themselves. Qualitative researchers in gerontology continue to draw inspiration from the early qualitative researchers cited above and others.[5,6]

Such early qualitative researchers' admonitions inspired my work on the nursing home experience in the early 1970s, for example, in which there was a need to be on the scenes of everyday life in a nursing facility to listen to how participants presented their lives and their care work "in their own words."[7] The aim of this work was to document and describe those lives and care work in terms that made sense to the participants themselves, according to the indigenous logics of their social worlds. "Being there" and listening to "their words" became my method of procedure, which also characterizes much of qualitative inquiry today.

Theoretical Complications

Things became more complicated, however, as qualitative researchers began to take serious heed of the conceptual and procedural choices they made as they put their methods to work. Not that early research shibboleths were dismissed or disappeared. Rather, in the final decades of the last century and into the new one, qualitative researchers started to pointedly question what it meant to "be there" or to consider what about subjects' "own" words was being captured when they were carefully listened to.

There was increased recognition that theoretical and methodological filters needed to be sorted out. What if not all of the forces that affected everyday life could be recognized through direct observation? What if talk and interaction— even in their own ostensible words—reproduced the experiential sensibilities of unacknowledged others, such as medical or pharmaceutical discourses of experience? If this were the case, then the context that affects everyday life, talk, and interaction was not transparent or readily accessible. Such critical concerns turned matters of method into theoretical, epistemological, and political, as well as procedural, concerns.[8-13] Qualitative methods were opened to reflexive, that is, self-aware and critical, consideration, informing researchers that the significance of the procedural imperatives of the early years needed to be figured in relation to epistemological assumptions.

In applying qualitative methods to aging, researchers can no longer simply put their best procedural foot forward. Looking carefully at social worlds is no longer as straightforward as it once seemed to be. Listening sympathetically to people has communicative and representational dimensions unknown to early qualitative researchers.[14] Qualitative methods today are immensely more conceptually sophisticated and researchers more analytically self-conscious than they had been. While being careful—being rigorous in data collection and analysis—is still important, rigor now has multiple conceptual horizons, which transforms the issue of being careful into something well beyond the technically procedural. Funding criteria and research oversight that ignore this development are themselves egregiously careless methodologically. The researcher's basic assumptions need to be questioned along with everything else.

Theorizing Method: Looking and Listening Beneath the Surface

Qualitative researchers today apply a broader range of techniques, which in part is a product of approaching method in theoretical as well as procedural terms. The early days were naturalistic, which meant that researchers tended to view the empirical world as a field of information to be discovered and analyzed. This (unwitting) orientation entailed systematically looking and listening in the context of people's lived experience, taking note of what was found, and reporting the results as accurately as possible. The idea was to present a true picture of the subject matter in view as completely and in as detailed a way as possible. Through their signature ethnographic fieldwork, anthropologists discovered and represented an amazing array of cultural patterns. Sociologists typically centered their attention on urban life, especially the city's problems, documenting the often unexpected ways the experiences of the "humbler classes," the city's "underlife," "vice areas," and other urban worlds were organized.

Look, see, discover, and report—these were the procedural bywords. True to these guidelines, social researchers opened our eyes to what were simply figured to be just "others" or just "over there." From peoples of Africa, Asia, Oceania, and North America to the gangs, slums, immigrants, and ethnic enclaves of American cities, anthropologists and sociologists conveyed amazingly nuanced accounts drawn from taking the time and putting forth the effort to actually enter into and experience the scenes and lives in question. Inspired by what anthropologist Clifford Geertz[15] refers to as "being there" and encouraged to write what sociologist John Van Maanen[16] calls "realist tales," these researchers produced many of the pioneering empirical studies of their disciplines. Detailed, rich and "thick" description painted vivid accounts of lives in these diverse places.

When We Look, What Do We See?

Today, available qualitative research methods are not this straightforward. While qualitative researchers continue to do fieldwork, conduct participant observation, and communicate directly with research participants, looking and listening have become as theoretical as they were once more or less procedural. One of the most compelling questions that led to the theorization of observational methods was "When we look, what do we see?" When my fieldwork at the pseudonymous Murray Manor first began in the early 1970s, the primary aim was to describe the facility as a small society, with its distinctive roles, rules, and relationships. Fieldwork at the Manor was designed to explore and document its way of life and social organization, something that hadn't been done before. While there were horror stories in newspapers and much anecdotal information about old age homes, a realist tale of social life that drew from systematic observation and careful documentation had yet to be written.

At the time, I was vaguely aware that important conceptual critiques of method had implications for what I assumed I was simply observing at the Manor. Initially, I figured the nursing home to be one organization, with various units, jobs, and types of clients of course, all more or less rationally configured under one institutional umbrella—in my case, Murray Manor, the nursing home. But I also was puzzled by the many claims and actions of participants that seemed reasonable to insiders and wholly unreasonable to outsiders. I began to entertain the idea that the reasonable and unreasonable were matters of perspective. The claims and actions of residents could seem so very unreasonable to front-line workers and vice-versa. The claims and actions of front-line workers could seem grossly unrealistic to administrative personnel and vice-versa. It became critical to question: What was being observed when these claims and actions unfolded before my very eyes? Conflicting parts of a whole? Angles of vision and the differential rhetorics lodged in a single organization? Perspective colored everything.

My view of the "whole" began to change mightily, along with my method of procedure, when I reconceptualized the whole into separate social worlds. With the ideas of Anselm Strauss,[17] Alfred Schutz,[18] Erving Goffman,[19] and Harold Garfinkel[20] whispering in the background, it was important to figure that what the Manor, its ostensible way of life, and its participants were for residents was envisioned differently than how it was envisioned for front-line workers, for example, or administrative personnel. Perhaps it was worth considering the idea that the Manor was a rather deceptive label for something significantly more complex, something less whole and unified than it seemed at the start. It became apparent that the observational units had to be framed in a different way and that it was not sufficient to carefully observe everyday life on the premises. It turned out that the study of one organization became research on three different social wholes located in one physical setting—top staff's world, the floor staff's world, and the world of the clientele.

Viewed in this way, what was being observed by me, especially at times when matters of being reasonable and unreasonable were at stake, was a collision of social worlds, not the reasonable or unreasonable claims or actions of individuals. The lenses of an initial, naturalistic method of procedure required refraction in different directions. Their optical strengths needed to be gauged separately, not in terms of some underlying organizational metric. Beginning with the understanding that my careful observations would reveal Murray Manor as a way of life led to a view that my careful observations were discovering the interplay of separate social worlds. The Manor simply wasn't one thing socially, but three. Methodologically, careful observation wasn't the issue, but it was rather what observation was understood to be viewing. The organizing framework suggested by this conceptual turnabout helped me make sense of what was being observed.

When We Listen, What Do We Hear?

The "theorization of method" centers both on *how* the material is collected as well as on *what* is collected. This theorization of method also draws from another compelling question: "When we listen, what do we hear?" Is good interviewing a matter of presenting unbiased and clear questions on the one side, and carefully recording the opinions of respondents on the other? Is good interviewing a matter of good interview technique, in other words? Who determines good interviewing technique, and if the technique is varied, how does it affect the results? For some interview researchers, listening actively and sympathetically to interviewees, especially being open to how the latter themselves frame questions and responses, provides a way of hearing the actual voices of those whose experience we wish to understand. In his important book *Research Interviewing*, Elliot Mishler[21] argues that putting this principle into practice "empowers" respondents to convey experience in their own terms. The question remains, however, where do those who are empowered in this way obtain the answers they provide to interviewers in such sympathetic circumstances? From where do they learn what they think, how they feel, and the meaning of what they've done or will do? (See Gubrium and Holstein 2002 for an extensive discussion of these issues.)

An Illustration of the Problem

Methodologically matured well beyond the early Murray Manor research days allowed me in the early 1980s to begin interview research with Alzheimer's disease (AD) sufferers, caregivers, and significant others with questions much like this in mind.[22] A distinctly reflexive view of method was in place to aid my observations and interviews with those who were engaged in what was eventually called the "Alzheimer's disease experience." Interviewing informed my ideas of the meaning of this experience from the varied perspectives of participants, while the ideas in turn provided resources for organizing the interview process. But the issue of what was being heard—the content—also was center stage, especially the question of what respondents were giving voice to when they spoke of their suffering, their burdens, and their professional practices. These were the days when the Alzheimer's disease movement was just getting off the ground. AD wasn't yet a commonly recognized disease category; other terms of reference such as "senility," "organic brain syndrome" (OBS), and "cerebro-vascular accident" (CVA) were standard usages for dementia in nursing homes and in geriatrics in general.

The methodological watershed for me came with a realization that the AD experience was as much a product of a *social movement* as it was given voice by individual participants. How they talked about their experiences reflected not only their experiences but something more. Not that older people, for example, weren't actually suffering from the consequences of an aging brain and its cognitive deficits. Rather, listening to my respondents—from the professionals to family caregivers, sufferers, and others—in terms of how the AD movement was shaping the meaning, and of course the moral contours, of what they were experiencing was critical. Listening carefully to how the knowledge and categories that the movement provided were playing into individual respondents' understanding of what was happening to them or to those they cared for turned my attention from personal knowledge to knowledge reproduction.

As the movement gained in strength, it appeared that what was being carefully heard in interview responses was the "voice" of the movement articulated through the "voice" of personal experience. Indeed, it became impossible to separate the two—and thus the idea of AD as an experiential project was born. The notion that both interview questions and responses could be part of a social movement suggested that my respondents weren't so much a sample of individuals as they were, in varying degrees, mouthpieces for a larger social form. The AD experience became a new frame of reference for an age-old set of cognitive and caregiving issues. This new frame of reference transformed the interview into something it could not have been as a method if it were individualistically conceived.[23] By listening to individuals' accounts, it became possible to hear how their concerns illustrated—or gave voice to—not only their own experience, but also to a socially significant social movement. (See Dorothy Smith[24] for an ethnographically oriented form of interviewing that draws from a construction of the voice of the subject linked with what she refers to as "relations of ruling.")

Representational Diversity: The Options for Describing Experience

How should peoples' experiences be depicted or represented? We have a diversity of choices, and the choices have moral implications. In reflecting on the proper way of representing subjects and their social worlds, Thomas and Znaniecki[3] (pp. 1846–1847) wrote, "We must put ourselves in the position of the subject who tries to find his way in this world, and we must remember, first of all, that the environment by which he is influenced and to which he adapts himself is his world, not the objective world of science." This view prompted these researchers to describe Poles' immigration experience through personal documents. (See Ken Plummer[25] for a discussion of the use of life documents for empirically engaging what he calls a "critical humanism.") They felt that letters written to, and received from, family members and others in Poland best represented what an immigrant goes through and what he or she thinks and feels as one way of life is displaced by another.

Much later, Goffman[26] proffered similar representational guidance related to the need to foreground the everyday social logic that shaped the lives and sentiments of those under consideration. By investigating the common features that linked different kinds of "total" institutions, he was able to show how the features of these organizations shaped the experiences of the "inmates." As if to say that our representational practices as researchers need to reflect the mundane contingencies of social worlds, Goffman offered a view of how to represent those worlds, "It was then and still is my belief that any group of persons—prisoners, primitives, pilots, or patients—develop a life of their own that becomes meaningful, reasonable, and normal once you get close to it, and that a good way to learn about any of these worlds is to submit oneself in the company of the members to the daily round of petty contingencies to which they are subject" (pp. ix–x).

From Thomas and Znaniecki to Goffman and others, the qualitative rule of thumb for representing members' social worlds has been to describe them as closely as possible to how they were experienced, unencumbered by the trappings of science. In other words, the rules, constraints, and other determining characteristics that structure peoples' lives need to be part of the analytic package. (This never meant that qualitative researchers weren't to be scientific, only that the mere trappings of science were no substitute for empirical truth. See Blumer,[27] Chapters 1, 7, 9, and 10.)

The Expansion of Options for Depicting Social Worlds

These sentiments still inform the representational practices of qualitative researchers. The contents of personal documents such as letters, diaries, files, and photograph albums continue to be featured in articles, book chapters, and monographs. Everyday talk and interaction in the settings we study are still part of qualitative researcher's representational stock-and-trade. What has changed is not that these are no longer featured in writing, but that there is diversity in how we depict or represent them.

The options for representing social worlds on their own terms have markedly expanded. The representational diversity of qualitative inquiry today has increased well beyond what it was in the early years. Postmodern sensibilities have encouraged some qualitative researchers to deconstructively feature their own textual practices alongside their research material as a way of highlighting, for example, the rhetorical meaning of Thomas and Znaniecki's, Goffman's, and others' naturalistic sentiments. These attempts to understand diverse accounts of experience have also led to the examination of the sometimes arbitrary division between researcher and subject.[1, 28-31] In all, these interpretations describe vivid ways of portraying the variety of meanings that are possible. Today, qualitative researchers borrow liberally from the representational practices of diverse disciplines to tell their stories. Many deliberately back away from scientistic (a belief that scientific language should always be weighted more heavily than other forms of representation) writing in order to convey the empirical truths in view.

Borrowing from the Humanities

One development has been the appropriation of representational practices more typical of the humanities to the task of describing lived experience. Carolyn Ellis and her associates[32,33] have featured a broad range of "alternative forms of qualitative writing." One alternative form that appears in their edited collections centers on Laurel Richardson's[34] work. Richardson uses poetry instead of prose to describe the circumstances of unwed mothers. In Richardson's view, sociological prose especially risks substituting scientistic language and argument for the terms and subjective understanding apparent in the in-depth interviews she conducted with these mothers. Richardson translates interview material into poems that, in her opinion, more truly convey the realities of the mothers' situations. Another alternative form of qualitative representation derives from theatre. Ellis and her partner Arthur Bochner (1992) write a play about Ellis's abortion experience, whose actual performance they argue is more realistic than reading a screenplay or an expository description would be. In both cases, the researcher's sense of getting close to the phenomenon in order to truthfully represent it goes beyond what mere words can convey, respectively to what poetry and performance reveal with words merely in tow.

Autoethnography

Another development that has led to representational diversity is autoethnography.[32,33,35] Many qualitative researchers have themselves undergone the experiences they study. Indeed, seasoned qualitative researchers encourage their students to start, if at all possible, with where they themselves have been. For example, Carol Rambo Ronai's[36] interest in the stigmatizing situations of childhood and young adulthood was prompted by her own stigmatizing experience of growing up with a mentally retarded parent. She also has written autoethnographic accounts of the experience of exotic dancers,[37] a world in which she was immersed as a young woman. In these accounts and in many others, such as autoethnographies of the lived experience of ostensible afflictions like bulimia,[38] qualitative researchers blur the boundaries between self and others as a way of diversely representing the interplay between inner lives and social worlds.[39]

Conclusion

In short, the array of qualitative methods of today comes out of a long tradition of epistemological debate and ferment. The methods do not exist apart from the theoretical frameworks and analytic concerns that spawned them. In considering qualitative methods today, two things are clear. One is that they are anything but a cafeteria of choices. Textbooks that survey the procedural waterfront in this way, reducing them to a set of cookbook methods, send the wrong message. Qualitative research techniques should not be viewed as a landscape in which one picks and chooses. All of these methods have now been reflexively challenged and appreciated for the forms of knowledge they provide and the kinds of empirical stories they construct. Qualitative researchers are no longer innocent epistemological bystanders to their craft. As we attempt to understand the aging experience as it relates to public health, we cannot proceed as if methods were simply, well, methods. This is because the method that is chosen comes from a theoretical tradition, the lens of which shapes the information that results.

A second thing that is clear today is that evaluating qualitative methodology solely for its technical proficiency fails to appreciate how profoundly moral it is. It is moral in that its leading mission has always been to represent forms of human experience on its own terms. It is now immensely more so as practitioners recognize that the substance and organization of the inner lives and social worlds they study connect in important ways with the kinds of questions practitioners put to the latter and the frameworks of understanding that lead them to apply specific methods in the first place. To pursue these questions at greater length requires a book. You are invited to read on.

Summary Points
- The researcher's methodology and theoretical stance provide a critical and determining lens that the researcher must acknowledge explicitly.
- Rigor has multiple conceptual horizons, including the reflexivity (self-awareness) of the researcher as well as the quality of data collection and analysis.
- Theorization of method focuses both on *how* the material is collected as well as on *what* is collected.
- Experience can be depicted or represented in a variety of ways, including through alternative forms of qualitative writing and autoethnography.

References

1) Gubrium, Jaber F. and James A. Holstein. *The New Language of Qualitative Method.* 1997; New York: Oxford University Press.
2) Mayhew, Henry. *London Labour and the London Poor,* Vol. 1. 1968; New York: Dover.
3) Thomas, W. I. and Florian Znaniecki. *The Polish Peasant in Europe and America.* 1974; New York: Octogon.
4) Whyte, William Foote. *Street Corner Society.* 1943; Chicago: University of Chicago Press.
5) Reinharz, Shulamit, and Graham Rowles (eds.). *Qualitative Gerontology.* 1988; New York: Springer.
6) Fry, Christine L. and Jennie Keith (eds.). *New Methods for Old Research.* 1980; Chicago: Center for Urban Policy, Loyola University.
7) Gubrium, Jaber F. *Living and Dying at Murray Manor.* 1975; New York: St. Martin's.
8) Gubrium, Jaber F. and David Silverman. *The Politics of Field Research.* 1989; London: Sage.
9) Cole, Thomas R., W. Andrew Achenbaum, Patricia L. Jakobi, and Robert Kastenbaum (eds.). *Voices and Vision of Aging: Toward a Critical Gerontology.* 1993; New York: Springer.
10) Hazan, Haim. *Old Age: Constructions and Deconstructions.* 1994; Cambridge: Cambridge University Press.
11) Featherstone, Mike and Andrew Wernick (eds.). *Images of Aging: Cultural Representations of Later Life.* 1995; London: Routledge.
12) Katz, Stephen. *Disciplining Old Age: The Formation of Gerontological Knowledge.* 1996; Charlottesville, VA: University of Virginia Press.
13) Andersson, Lars (eds.). *Cultural Gerontology.* 2002; Westport, CT: Auburn House.
14) Gubrium, Jaber F. and James A. Holstein (eds.). *Handbook of Interview Research.* 2002; Thousand Oaks, CA: Sage.
15) Geertz, Clifford. *Works and Lives: The Anthropologist as Author.* 1988; Stanford: Stanford University Press.
16) Van Maanen, John. *Tales of the Field: On Writing Ethnography.* 1988; Chicago: University of Chicago Press.
17) Strauss, Anselm L. *Mirrors and Masks: The Search for Identity.* 1959; New York: Free Press.
18) Schutz, Alfred. *The Phenomenology of the Social World.* 1967; Chicago: Northwestern University Press.
19) Goffman, Erving. *The Presentation of Self in Everyday Life.* 1959; New York: Doubleday.
20) Garfinkel, Harold. *Studies in Ethnomethodology.* 1967; Englewood Cliffs, NJ: Prentice-Hall.
21) Mishler, Elliot G. *Research Interviewing: Context and Narrative.* 1986; Cambridge: Harvard University Press.
22) Gubrium, Jaber F. *Oldtimers and Alzheimer's: The Descriptive Organization of Senility.* 1986; Greenwich, CT: JAI Press.
23) Holstein, James A. and Jaber F. Gubrium. *The Active Interview.* 1995; Thousand Oaks, CA: Sage.
24) Smith, Dorothy E. *The Everyday World as Problematic: A Feminist Sociology.* 1987; Boston: Northeastern University Press.
25) Plummer, Ken. *Documents of Life 2.* 2001; London: Sage.
26) Goffman, Erving. *Asylums.* Garden City, 1961; New York: Doubleday.
27) Blumer, Herbert. *Symbolic Interaction: Perspective and Method.* 1969; Englewood Cliffs, NJ: Prentice-Hall.

28) Clifford, James and George E. Marcus (eds.). *Writing Culture.* 1986; Berkeley, CA: University of California Press.

29) Atkinson, Paul. *The Ethnographic Imagination.* 1990; London: Routledge.

30) Denzin, Norman K. *Images of Postmodern Society.* 1991; London: Sage.

31) Clough, Patricia Ticineto. *The End(s) of Ethnography.* 1992; Thousand Oaks, CA: Sage.

32) Ellis, Carolyn and Michael G. Flaherty (eds.). *Investigating Subjectivity: Research on Lived Experience.* 1992; Thousand Oaks, CA: Sage.

33) Ellis, Carolyn and Arthur Bochner P. (eds.). *Composing Ethnography: Alternative Forms of Qualitative Writing.* 1996; Walnut Creek, CA: AltaMira Press.

34) Richardson, Laurel. "The Consequences of Poetic Representation: Writing the Other, Rewriting the Self." pp. 125-140 in *Investigating Subjectivity,* Carolyn Ellis and Michael G. Flaherty (eds.). 1992; Thousand Oaks, CA: Sage.

35) Reed-Danahay, Deborah E. *Auto/Ethnography: Rewriting the Self and the Social.* 1997; New York: Berg.

36) Rambo Ronai, Carol. "My Mother is Mentally Retarded." pp. 109-131 in *Composing Ethnography,* Carolyn Ellis and Arthur P. Bochner (eds.). 1996; Thousand Oaks, CA: AltaMira.

37) Rambo Ronai, Carol. "The Reflexive Self Through Narrative: A Night in the Life of an Exotic Dancer/Researcher." Pp. 102-124 in *Investigating Subjectivity,* Carolyn Ellis and Michael G. Flaherty (eds.). 1992; Thousand Oaks, CA: Sage.

38) Tillman, Healy, Lisa M. "A Secret Life in a Culture of Thinness: Reflections on Body, Food, and Bulimia." pp. 76-108 in *Composing Ethnography,* Carolyn Ellis and Arthur P. Bochner (eds.). 1996; Walnut Creek, CA: AltaMira.

39) Holstein, James A. and Jaber F. Gubrium (eds.). *Inner Lives and Social Worlds.* 2003; New York: Oxford University Press.

Chapter 3

Cultural Forces in the Acceptance of Qualitative Research: Advancing Mixed Method Research

Mark Luborsky, PhD and Andrea Sankar, PhD

Introduction:
The Riddle of Acceptance of Qualitative Research

The Riddle. Are qualitative methods not accepted in research in aging? While the abiding sense of embattlement over qualitative methods in gerontology is a riddle, it also provides a salient cultural context for its conduct. Even when decried as "unproductive"[1] and "smoke and mirrors,"[2] and obituaries of the debate are offered,[3] the discourse nonetheless endures; often, researchers who share qualitative interests talk about these tensions in formal and informal conversations.

While qualitative researchers pay attention to the contexts of the research phenomena and processes, relatively little formal attention is directed toward the socio-cultural settings in which qualitative research itself is proposed and reported. This neglect may contribute to the argument over the utility of qualitative methods. This chapter therefore examines the societal contexts in which qualitative research is conducted as a way of advancing the field and providing answers.

The other articles in this volume offer valuable details and insights about conceptual and methodological considerations in performing qualitative and mixed qualitative and quantitative methods research. The goal of this chapter is to characterize the larger contemporary contexts of qualitative research. Indeed the plethora of specialty journals, handbooks, and articles suggests that rather than being a new cutting edge approach, qualitative research is well into middle age.

A Cultural Context for Qualitative Research is Needed

Culturally literate qualitative researchers must develop an appreciative attitude[4,5] toward the 'contextual' features of their scientific community in addition to learning about the diverse lives and stories of the persons they study. Not only must they master the techniques of qualitative inquiry but they must be able to grasp the social contexts underpinning the methodology. Therefore, we propose using the lens of "communities of practice"[6,7] to ascertain the scientific paradigms behind the methods. For example, Agar and McDonald[8] identify endemic flaws in focus group content analyses that are due to "cutting and pasting" quotes without context. This practice greatly limits the utility of quotes, and the authors suggest how to provide the necessary context. In short, simply translating methods across disciplines and specifying the qualitative analog to quantitative design issues will not dissolve the cultural factors that underlie concerns about qualitative methods. In addition, skillful attention to the cultural factors in the wider community of research practice is needed.

The value of qualitative research is clear. Qualitative research has long made significant contributions to knowledge about aging, human development and the conditions of living in old age that span basic discovery to the evaluation of intervention outcomes. Qualitative methods complement and expand gerontology's ability to understand a wider range of phenomena than is possible using quantitative or diagnostic methods alone.

The history of gerontology reveals many examples of such key contributions. Ory and Williams,[9] for example, reviewed the history of projects funded by the National Institute of Aging (NIA) about rehabilitation. Rehabilitation is a relatively new discipline that enables people to regain functional ability and restore participation in meaningful roles and identities[10,33] instead of accepting stereotypes of old age as decay, disability, suffering and neglect. This review highlighted the sequence of NIA's projects on several disabling chronic later life conditions once accepted as normal and not treatable, such as incontinence, hip fracture, and stroke. Today as a result of such advances, geriatric rehabilitation is no longer an oxymoron.[9,11] Ory and Williams[9] traced how the first projects funded were qualitative discovery-oriented studies designed to map out the salient issues and characterize key factors and measurement strategies. Subsequent studies used qualitative and standardized methods to assess the relative contribution of these to desired and undesirable outcomes. Lastly, building on both qualitative and quantitative knowledge, other researchers created interventions to reduce these forms of human distress and improve the experience of living into older age.

For example, ageist stereotypes that considered urinary incontinence as a "nuisance" meant that it was once ignored. Qualitative methods of ethnographic research helped dispel the stereotype. Mitteness and Barker [12] documented that institutionalized elderly endured embarrassment and discomfort because staff used diapers rather than checked for alternative causes, such as infections or bladder muscle weakness. Later studies found treatable causes and developed effective therapies. Today, rather than endure social and physical discomfort, pelvic floor muscle exercises, surgery, and medications are routinely prescribed, and incontinence rates are far lower.

Qualitative methods are well suited to discovering and interpreting cultural diversity and social disparity in health and aging for several reasons briefly outlined here.

First, qualitative methods are designed to identify and interpret issues regarding culture and group specific meanings and values. The methods are suited to discovery, description and interpretation of diverse ways of life, values and meanings, and the complexities of pluralistic social systems. They capture the distinctive language, concepts, worldviews, patterns of social relationships, and behaviors that are not adequately grasped by existing standardized measures and categories. Qualitative methods further contribute by identifying the appropriate basic units of analyses including, for example, indigenous concepts of the family, identity and roles, community, or meaningful quality of life. Some of these concepts can be converted to structured measures. Yet other kinds of knowledge and experience, such as histories, or those embodied in narrative forms of reasoning or symbolic forms, are not reducible to standardized measures and require qualitative methods.

Second, qualitative methods can enhance rapport and trust among participants since they often collaborate to define relevant topics, issues, and perspectives, and to express views and experiences in their own words. As a result, the credibility of the information is stronger and the results and recommendations may gain wider acceptance in the community under study.

That being said, we must ask why forms of knowledge such as statistical and epidemiological data are regarded as more authoritative than stories and case studies *despite these significant qualitative contributions* over the years. Notwithstanding published recognized guidelines for qualitative studies [13–16] that provide validation by specifying scientific criteria for the proper review of qualitative research and the numerous qualitative journals and books on knowledge and literature on methods,[17] the scholarly discourse in gerontology continues to reflect friction and doubt around the value of qualitative research.

The task for qualitative researchers is to *enhance the credibility and vigor of qualitative methods in order to assure that valuable findings from qualitative work are accepted more widely* among the community of scientists. The time is ripe to ask two questions: (1) What can we learn from consideration of the cultural contexts of qualitative research itself to help understand the tension, and (2) how can we redress the enduring issues raised about such work? The adept qualitative researcher must be aware of and respond to the signs and practices that are accepted as markers of useful, good new knowledge building tools.*

Answers to these questions offer at least two contributions. First, if we are to realize the potential of qualitative research, we need to understand the cultural contexts for research methods which aid or impede their effective use. Second, qualitative researchers should focus on improving the scientific rigor and credibility of methods—as opposed to criticizing quantitative research.

In the following sections we outline an ethnographic perspective on the tension from the perspective of doing and reviewing qualitative studies and proposals. We review the debate within the scholarly research community in order to highlight potentially valuable avenues to diminish this unproductive dynamic.

---

*While others have argued for methodological pragmatism (Patton)[3] and independent qualitative research evaluation criteria (Cicourel[18]; Denzin and Lincoln[19]; Lincoln and Gupta[20]), the focus here is on the wider settings and communities of practice of that knowledge production.

The Debate of Qualitative versus Quantitative Discourse

Where Do We Find This Debate in Scientific Exploration?

One might be surprised to know that qualitative methods are deeply inscribed in the knowledge building practices of many scientific communities including mathematics, chemistry, physics, and biology. These fields select qualitative or quantitative methods to develop understanding suited to the particular phenomena or stages in knowledge development. For example, Richard Feynman,[21] a 1965 Nobel Laureate in Physics, declares himself a qualitative researcher who hopes to someday achieve quantitative stages in his inquiries. Given the centrality of qualitative methods in these fields, it is thus instructive to ask why the tension is more vociferous in gerontology and social sciences than in other disciplines.

Language differentiating qualitative and quantitative research tasks is evident in technological projects such as outer space missions to Mars and the moon or inner space mapping of the human genome and the contexts of daily life as well as in behavioral and social science. NASA's Mars mission to explore and gain knowledge about the unique and shared origins of bodies in the universe used qualitative and quantitative techniques in its research. After touchdown the Mars Lander extended its "probe" to qualitatively question the surface by opening up a scoop to collect "samples" of the surface; it then conducted qualitative chemical analyses in order to identify and describe the kinds of elements in the soil. These basic discoveries answered many burning questions about the basic nature of Mars. Next, using quantitative methods from chemistry and physics, the samples were analyzed to learn how the elements combined into compounds and their relative distribution in the area.

This vivid lesson from NASA teaches that qualitative and mixed methods are important tools for terrestrial and interplanetary research. It reminds that one must not equate nor limit the technology of computer hardware or software with one kind of research question and method. Sound scholarship about Mars as well as about people on Earth requires the proper mix of methods designed for the research question.

Further, an ethnographic glance at the titles of standard texts from *Vogel's Qualitative Inorganic Analysis*[22] to *General Chemistry with Qualitative Analyses*[23] to genomic analyses by engineers [24] reveals a scientific reliance on the qualitative. Cell biologists use the language of "high-content analyses" to describe new stem cell research (e.g., Giuliano et al. 2003).[25] Competence in both qualitative and quantitative approaches is integral. Qualitative methods help determine the basic kinds of elements, molecules, or atoms that are present (whether in a test tube or a sample scooped up by a remotely operated probe) while quantitative methods serve to answer questions about what proportion of those elements are there and how they are combined.

Qualitative methods in general help discover salient things to measure and help describe their basic form when information about them is limited. The second major reason qualitative research is needed is to better characterize certain phenomena that are not adequately captured by existing tools. The history of a group, profession, or individual lifetime can not readily be reduced to a series of structured questions or medical diagnostic classifications. Certain forms of experience and knowledge are only conveyed through narratives and are not reducible to standardized question-reply formats. And yet they have a powerful and enduring influence as these represent groups or persons' guiding sense of where they have come from, what their life is like today, and importantly, their expectations for the future.

Why Does the Debate About the Value of Qualitative Methods Endure?

No one argues for the value of qualitative chemistry over quantitative chemistry. Why does this debate in the social sciences still arise? A few brief speculations about the sources for the dissension over methods in gerontology can be offered.

Perhaps the dissensions are due to the multidisciplinarity of gerontology required by the multidimensional phenomena of aging. Gerontology draws from diverse fields and methods to answer complex questions about aging. Thus, it fosters a rich interface similar to the ecologically rich intertidal zone, where the hard land and fluid sea of positivist, social science, and interpretive epistemologies meet in a continual ebb and flow. Perhaps mutual respect as well as misunderstanding across disciplinary languages is therefore inevitable.

Perhaps too, as scholars have noted,[13,14,26–28] a confounding of epistemological and ontological issues may underlie the tension. Epistemology concerns the sources and limits of our knowledge including how and what we can know about a phenomenon[29] whereas ontology is about learning what actually exists or is true. We argue that the language and structure of qualitative research is identifiably 'liberal" and taps basic social tensions in our society. Agar[30] labels these "rich points" of cultural contention. For example, qualitative research seeks to bring out the "voices of the people" and express pluralism through the discovery of multiple and alternative histories.[31] Such research reveals counter-narratives by clarifying each individual's own ideas and ways of understanding that are separate from socially normative categories. It discovers and respects "diversity" and helps to identify oppressive power structures which disempower some groups and privilege others.

At the level of research design, projects are collaboratively guided by sharing power with the study participants, significantly called "informants" rather than "subjects," and are not controlled authoritatively by the researcher. The designs are more open and fluid rather than traditionally fixed and predetermined. Reinharz and Rowles[32] further note how methods may be gendered: quantitative methods are considered male and qualitative methods are female. Following this line of argument, the differing professional languages and choices of methodologies can be seen as evoking contested political traditions in the society beyond the realm of the "scientific" study. Perhaps, resistance to qualitative methods or findings in gerontology stems from such unrecognized value-laden principles. Understanding the values implicit in science is one way to see the contexts shaping the practices in a scientific community.

Terms and Tools in the Practice of Qualitative Research

Methods as Tools

Humans create and use tools to apprehend and fashion the environment and conditions of life. While our tools shape the world, they also profoundly shape our perception of things we have come to take for granted. For example, the telephone, the Internet, the automobile, and the bicycle shape what we define as "near" and "far," while medicine defines expectable comfort and life span. Relevant to the qualitative debate is that the research tools we use also associate us with a particular social group, just as the tools we use for eating (forks, fingers, or chop sticks) signal a particular cultural identity and heritage.

Similarly, qualitative methods are tools that carve and fashion certain forms of data and understandings. Some tools are intentionally crude so as to allow for wider latitude in the forms of information, scale, scope, and size that can be produced from them. Other qualitative methods can be viewed as more sophisticated given the rapid advances in methods and critical understandings. For example, it is no longer sufficient to describe a research plan as "using qualitative methods or analyses" without specifying the particular kinds of methods, settings, and how they will be conducted in light of their recognized strengths and limits. Similarly, technology and qualitative research converge as computer software now enables greater efficiency, systematicity, replicability, and sample size than imaginable by early researchers.

By using qualitative methods alone or in combination with other paradigms, we aim to contribute to gerontology's knowledge base. In multidisciplinary settings (or in the tidal boundary zones described above) the boundaries of disciplines comprise a rich environment that yields discoveries. Mixed methods promise findings beyond those that derive from a single tradition. Using a combination of methods, however, must require attention to the diverse demands, restrictions, and norms of the collaborating disciplines than when working in a single methodology.

Mixed methods collaboration is not so readily actualized in practice for a variety of reasons. Sometimes there is a great distance between the quantitative and qualitative camps in gerontology. The languages used by each reveal a window into social worlds and realms of meanings. A brief examination of the language of scientific practice examined below will help provide a second main sensitizing concept for the practices of mixed methods in current social science.

The Hidden Meanings of Tools and Design Criteria

The key terms used to design and evaluate research such as power, reliability, validity, control, and independent and dependent factors are tools with a double life.[10,33,34] While their surface meanings are listed in the dictionary, they carry symbolic connotations that are extremely value laden. They are like a set of precepts for a proper and just society, such as those embodied in the Ways of Tao, the Q'ran, or the biblical Ten Commandments. Researchers have a set of precepts and ritual specialists called "statisticians" who are consulted for guidance in the design and repair of projects. We know that the current definition of a "representative" sample is distributed across a range of social settings, from scientific journals to legislative debates about political districts and representation, to sampler boxes of chocolate. In daily life socially normative expectations for child and adult development focus on predetermined criteria in growth and achievement, such as personal independence, dependence, control, and reliability, and these are culturally relative. At the group level we see the same criteria and employ a cadre of specialists, such as rehabilitation and psychological therapists.

The language of science subtly expresses cultural values, and we must be attuned to these meanings. The deeper moral vein in our work is revealed when we are instructed early on to construct and carefully protect "independent" and "dependent" variables and the statistical "power" of our designs. We "control" variables and enhance peoples' sense of control. We are taught to judge and describe constructs in terms of "valid" or "invalid." (The latter word also denotes disability.) Attention to power issues (inadequate or excessive) is pervasive from government, politics, and military, to interpersonal relationships. We want to assure adequate power in machines to perform their function. It is important to be alert to these associations and meanings in scholarship.

Basic constructs, such as independence, stress, family, frailty, and self, are cultural concepts commonly applied in gerontology that are not value-free or absolute variables. Culture patterns our knowledge by way of the basic building blocks of science. We seldom devote attention to how knowledge embodies our cultural world-views, and we treat variables and scientific procedures as value-free when they are not. The analytic constructs bring cultural assumptions about the work into the discipline's history and the research process, as Moss and Moss[35] document in the case of the disenfranchisement of death and grief from mainstream gerontology (see also Achenbaum,[36] Cole,[37] and Estes and Binney[38]). Less explicitly, the constructs also carry with them an implicit teleology for maintaining society and individual development that replicate current values, social roles, and inter-group structures. A good example of this is how Cohen and Sokolovsky[39] describe how the dire conditions faced by older men in the Bowery are defined by individual adjustment problems rather than by the societal and political factors that create the problems.

The consensus of a scholarly community defines objective "reality" and informs some fundamental quantitative norms, such as calculations for statistical consensus. For example, calculations of statistical power specify a convention of an agreed upon acceptable level of indeterminacy and likelihood, given the number of informants, variables, and effect sizes. A study designed to provide 80 percent power, defining a "medium effect size," thus allows for a determination of statistical significance with up to 20 percent of the phenomena or behavior not fitting the pattern. These social constructions of reality should be familiar to qualitative researchers.

A Constructive Stance for Qualitative Research

Research design constructs (such as sample, power, and independence) are tools that help achieve valued core cultural ideals. These socially conventional practices enable us to build knowledge that is culturally defined as acceptable and desired. Even more significantly, concern about the adequacy of concepts such as power, representativeness, independence, and dependence, pervade our ideas about good society, not just research. By developing a critical orientation and an appreciative attitude to such cultural factors in the community of multidisciplinary research, qualitative researchers can identify those issues as productive opportunities rather than unachievable expectations that disproportionately disadvantage them. Thus, the qualitative researcher can choose to alter his/her stance to attend to sample, power, or other design features. The critiques should be understood as concerns about not attending to shared community values and criteria that are considered basic building blocks for research and for individual and group social life.

The noted philosopher of science, Karl Popper, wrote that in the conduct of scientific inquiry it is rarely possible to achieve the ideal, and systematic approaches to identify and remedy the intrinsic biases, errors, and missteps that bedevil achieving new truths are needed[29]. Stated differently, the research design ideals command attention because they are difficult to achieve. Accomplishing an acceptable level of power, control, and independence among variables is a goal rather than an absolute state. The scholarly community recognizes the inevitability of limitations and flaws and is eager to learn how a particular study has attempted to overcome rather then evade them.

Therefore, sensitivity to the cultural underpinning of the terms used in qualitative research suggests why neglecting the concerns of quantitative and positivistic traditions evokes strong reactions, including lack of recognition, acceptance, and exclusion. Indeed, such strong proscriptions are as predictable as if one ignored the speed or traffic signal conventions of a community. Further, penalties are more severe when one evades the officer enforcing the community standards for safe driving. Thus when preparing for the reviewers who evaluate submissions for conference papers, journal articles, and grant proposals, this caution should be kept well in mind.

Conclusion

No particular methodological approach is without limitations or consequences. If we want research findings to have an impact, our task is to help readers and reviewers understand the multiplicity of approaches and their relevance to particular problems. While some approaches are more palatable to the positivistic and quantitative approach of mainstream public health and medical institutions, such as the National Institutes of Health, reviewers are less biased against any one method than an incompletely specified proposal or article.[13] The researcher must demonstrate accountability and defend the usefulness of methods for achieving the goal. Critiques offered by quantitative researchers should be carefully considered and fully responded to, rather than dismissed as unfounded criticism of a paradigm or discipline. Major public scientific institutions such as NIH and NSF have identified the under-specification of methods and research design as the single most significant flaw in the qualitative research proposals submitted for review. Therefore, we argue in this chapter that qualitative researchers must understand how the language and practices of their research are perceived as fundamental tools with cultural connotations and identifications.

Quantitative researchers are exquisitely aware that their best methods only approximate the reality they seek to understand and must attend to potential bias and lack of power. They may wonder why qualitative researchers do not appear to share their concern about the reliability of the data or potential biases in the sample if the researchers do not address such issues. Failure to appreciate this concern limits how qualitative research insights and findings can be effectively disseminated and socially legitimated. Ignoring the context of this kind of critique also stunts potential advances in research that are needed to better understand the nature and forms of human social life and experiences of health, aging, and development over the life course and in later life. Qualitative researchers who defend their approach might redirect their energies toward the refinement and critical evaluation of qualitative methods themselves, and how to understand better the social and cultural contexts in which the particular methods used to derive the findings will be interpreted.

Our hope is that we can achieve the larger purpose of gerontology by enhancing the acceptability of findings derived from qualitative research. That goal can be pursued more effectively by keeping considerations about the epistemological and cultural features of qualitative research that have been raised in this chapter clearly in mind. Multiple methods are vitally needed to appreciate and address the spectrum of issues confronting the growing numbers of elderly and their profound influences across societies. Attention to these issues will help produce strong research that helps answer these questions.

Summary Points
- We ask why the value of qualitative methods is still seen to be an issue among researchers in aging.
- Knowledge of the scientific rationale and social connotations for each methodology is needed in addition to mastery of the methods.
- The history of gerontology reveals the meaningful contributions of qualitative methods.
- "Hard" science often uses qualitative as well as quantitative methods.
- Qualitative researchers should improve the nuts and bolts of doing and refining their methods.
- Qualitative methods help us discover salient things to measure and to characterize certain phenomena that are not adequately captured by existing tools.
- Qualitative researchers must learn to answer questions such as reliability and validity in order to be taken seriously.

References

1) Miles, M. and Huberman, A. *Qualitative Data Analysis*, 2nd Ed. 1994; Newbury Park, CA: Sage

2) Schmuttermaier, J. and Schmitt, D. Smoke and Mirrors: Modernist Illusions in the Quantitative versus Qualitative Research Debate. 2001; *Sociological Research Online,* 2001; 6(2). www.socresonline.org.uk/6/2/schmuttermaier.html

3) Patton, M. *Utilization-Focused Evaluation.* 1997; Thousand Oaks, CA: Sage.

4) Schafer, R. The Appreciative Attitude and the Construction of Multiple Histories. *Psychoanalysis and Contemporary Thought,* 1979; 2:3-24.

5) Schafer, R. *Narrative Actions in Psychoanalysis: Narratives of Space and Narratives of Time.* 1981; Worcester, MA: Clark University.

6) Wenger, E. *Communities of Practice,* 1998, New York; Cambridge University Press

7) Lave, J. and Wenger, E., *Situated Learning: Legitimate Peripheral Participation,* 1991. New York; Cambridge University..

8) Agar, M. and MacDonald, J. Focus Groups and Ethnography. *Human Organization* 1995; 54(l):78-86.

9) Ory, M. and Williams, T.F. Rehabilitation: Small Goals, Sustained Interventions. *Annals American Academy of Political and Social Science,* 1990; 503:661-76.

10) Luborsky, M. The Cultural Adversity of Physical Disability: Erosion of Full Adult personhood. *Journal of Aging Studies.* 1994b; 8(3):239-253.

11) Brody, S. and Ruff, G. *Aging and Rehabilitation.* 1986; New York: Springer.

12) Mitteness, L., Barker, J. Stigmatizing a "Normal" Condition: Urinary Incontinence in Late Life. *Medical Anthropology Quarterly.* 1995; 9:188-210.

13) National Institute of Health, *Qualitative Methods in Health Research: Opportunities and Considerations in Application and Review.* 2001; NIH Publication No. 02-5046 Bethesda MD.

14) National Science Foundation. *Workshop on Interdisciplinary Standards for Systematic Qualitative Research.* National Science Foundation, 2004; Available at: http://www.wjh.harvard.edu/nsfqual/

15) Ragin, C,, Nagel, J., and White, P. Workshop on Scientific Foundations of Qualitative Research. 2004; National Science Foundation. Available at: http://www.nsf.gov/pubs/2004/nsf04219/nsf04219_1.pdf

16) Frechtling, J. and Sharp, L. (eds.). *User-Friendly Handbook for Mixed Method Evaluations.* 1997; National Science Foundation. Publication NSF97-153

17) Patton, M. Two Decades of Developments in Qualitative Inquiry. *Qualitative Social Work.* 2002; 1(3): 261-283.

18) Cicourel, A. *Method and Measurement in Sociology.* 1964; New York: Free Press of Glencoe.

19) Denzin, N., and Lincoln, Y. *Handbook of Qualitative Research, 2nd Ed.,* 2000; Thousand Oaks, California: Sage.

20) Lincoln, Y., Guba, E. *Naturalistic Inquiry.* 1985; Beverly Hills: Sage.

21) Feynman, R. *The Pleasure in Finding Things Out.* 1999; Helix Books/Perseus Books, 1999.

22) Svehla, G. *Vogel's Qualitative Inorganic Analysis 7th Edition.* 1986; New Jersey: Prentice Hall.

23) Holtzelaw, H. F. Jr., Robinson, W., Odom, J., and Holtzelaw, H. F. *General Chemistry with Qualitative Analysis—10th Edition.* 1996; Houghton Mifflin Company.

24) Peleg, M., Gabashvili, I., and Altman, R. Qualitative Models of Molecular Function: Linking Genetic Polymorphisms of tRNA to Their Functional Sequelae. *Proceedings Of The IEEE,* 2002; 90(12):1875-1886.

25) Giuliano, K., Haskins, J., and Taylor, D. Advances in High Content Screening for Drug Discovery. *Assay and Drug Development Technologies*. 2003; 1(4):565-577.

26) Ragin, C., Becker, H. (eds). *What is a Case? Exploring Foundations of Sociological Inquiry*. 1995; New York: Cambridge University Press.

27) Devers, K. How Will We Know "Good" Qualitative Research When We See It? Beginning the Dialogue in Health Services Research. *Health Services Research*, 1999; 34(5):1153

28) Ragin, C., Nagel, J., and White, P. *Proceedings of the Workshop on the Scientific Foundations of Qualitative Research Workshop*, Publication #04219. National Science Foundation, 2003; Arlington, VA. Available at: http://www.nsf.gov/publications/pub_summ.jsp?ods_key=nsf04219

29) Popper, K. *Conjectures and Refutations: The Growth of Scientific Knowledge*. 1963; London: Routledge Kegan Paul.

30) Agar, M. *Language Shock: Understanding the Culture of Conversation*. 1994; New York, Wm. Morrow

31) Zinn, H. *A People's History of the United States*. 1980; New York: Harper and Row Publishers.

32) Reinharz , S. and Rowles, G.D. 1988; *Qualitative Gerontology*. New York: Springer.

33) Luborsky, M. The Identification of Themes and Patterns. In J. Gubrium, A. Sankar (eds.), *Qualitative Methods in Aging Research*. 1994a; New York: Sage Publications.

34) Luborsky, M., and Rubinstein, R. Sampling in Qualitative Research: Rationale, Issues, and Methods. *Research on Aging* 1995; 17(1):89-113.

35) Moss, M. and Moss, S. Death of the very old. In K. Doka (Ed), *Disenfranchised Grief: Recognizing Hidden Sorrow*. 1989; Lexington, MA: Lexington Books.

36) Achenbaum, A. *Old Age in a New Land*. 1978; Baltimore: Johns Hopkins University.

37) Cole, T. *What Does it Mean to Grow Old: Reflections from the Humanities*. 1986; Durham, NC: Duke University

38) Estes, C. and Binney, E. The Biomedicalization of Aging: Dangers and Dilemmas. *The Gerontologist*, 1990; 29, 587-597.

39) Cohen, C. and Sokolovsky, J. *Old Men of the Bowery: Strategies for Survival Among the Homeless*. 1989; New York: Guilford.

Chapter 4

Qualitative Data Collection for Aging Research:
Choosing the Right Method

Shoshanna Sofaer, DrPH.

Introduction

In part because of the diverse disciplinary and theoretical roots of qualitative research, a wide range of data collection methods is available for use within this tradition. Further, many who use qualitative methods combine them with quantitative approaches. Even within each broad data collection method, the researcher can choose among multiple variations on the basic theme. This chapter therefore explores two questions: 1) What is the range of qualitative data collection methods available for the field of aging research? and 2) What is at stake in making decisions about both the general method and the specific variation to be used? The term "explore" is used advisedly, because there is not (and perhaps should not be) a set of hard and fast rules to apply. As with so many decisions in the research enterprise, judgment based on in-depth knowledge of highly "local" circumstances must be applied. Since the work and premise of qualitative researchers may be viewed with skepticism by single-minded quantitative researchers, it is necessary to clearly articulate the rationale for data collection choices in proposals for research support and manuscripts submitted for publication.

In exploring the questions noted above, this chapter will offer real and hypothetical examples to illustrate the use of methods "on the ground." In closing, we will identify a brief methodological research agenda to help answer puzzling questions that recur when making methodological choices in aging research, especially when exploring the increasing diversity of the aging population.

The Range of Qualitative Data Collection Methods

There are three primary data collection methods in qualitative research: interviews, focus groups, and observation.

Interviews

Within the broad category of interviews there are two major types, one far more common than the other. The more common type is the "key informant interview." The one element that all key informant interviews should have in common is that they depend on open-ended questions.[1,2] Indeed, the open ended approach to data collection is inherently qualitative in nature, in contrast to surveys where questions are closed-ended and provide responses that can easily be "counted." The use of the term "key" informant implies that the respondent has been chosen because she/he has knowledge, holds a position, or has had experiences that are of interest to the researcher.

A less common type of qualitative interview is the "cognitive" interview.[3,4] These interviews are designed to elicit from respondents their understanding and interpretation, and sometimes their reaction to, some kind of stimulus material. The term "cognitive" implies that the primary goal is to understand the mental processes by which people deal with material. This approach developed as a technique for testing items in surveys and is now considered a major methodological advance over what used to be called "pre-testing." In the original use, people similar to those in the survey sampling frame answer a set of survey items. Either concurrently or afterwards, they are asked open-ended questions to explore whether they understood the items and response options as the surveyor intended, and the cognitive process that led them to answer a particular question in the way they did. This method is now also used in the formative testing of information materials of all kinds, and helps ensure that people like those in the target audience for the materials understand them as intended.[5] The interviews also help clarify whether the materials provide the desired level of detail and whether they may be considered engaging, offensive, or elicit other reactions.

Dimensions of variation in the collection of interview data. There are four major dimensions of variation in the design of interviews:

1) How much structure is involved?

2) How many participants are involved in either doing the interview or in being interviewed?

3) What is the mode of administration?

4) Is there a "stimulus" in addition to the questions that are used during the interview process?

Structure

Cognitive interviews are inherently quite structured since they are designed to learn about responses to a specific stimulus. The extent of structure in a key informant interview varies along a continuum from entirely unstructured to highly structured. Many interviews are best described as semi-structured.

What does structure entail as a dimension of variation in interviews? First, the extent of formality in identifying respondents can vary considerably. For example, in ethnographic research[6] the researcher is most likely to enter a field setting in as unobtrusive and natural a manner as possible, and then select people to interview who happen to be in the setting at the time(s) the researcher is present. He/she can select people to interview based on specific characteristics of interest or the selection can be more random or opportune (though it is important to note that the randomness in this case is not designed to produce a probability sample). A second aspect of structure is whether the questions to be asked have been thought through and written ahead of time. In some cases, an "interview protocol" may amount to little more than a listing of topics. To remain as unobtrusive as possible, the researcher may memorize the topics rather than carry a list into the field setting. In other cases, each question is carefully word-smithed, as in the design of a closed-ended survey instrument, and questions are to be asked exactly as worded. The more common intermediate design is the semi-structured interview, in which carefully worded questions are made available in a protocol; the interviewer is expected to use his or her judgment to reword questions as needed, depending on respondent characteristics, prior statements, or indications that the respondent does not fully understand the question. Furthermore, in the context of semi-structured interviews, the researcher may, upon hearing an unexpected response, come up with an entirely new and different question that had not been included earlier.

A related issue is whether questions are asked in a particular sequence. Question sequences are rigidly adhered to only in the most structured interviews. A pre-determined sequence is generally alien to unstructured interviews. While a sequence is typically incorporated into a written protocol in semi-structured interviews, the researcher is nonetheless free to change the sequence. For example, a respondent may begin to answer a question or raise an issue addressed later in the protocol. In all but the most highly structured interviews the interviewer will have the option of either jumping ahead to the relevant set of questions, or asking the respondent to "hold that thought" because the topic will come up later on.

Common elements of qualitative interviews are "probes." With probing, an inherent part of unstructured interviews, the researcher follows the lead of the respondent and uses related questions to elicit additional detail or nuance. Probing can be done quite spontaneously in semi-structured interviews, as well. However, for different reasons, probes are often written into interview protocols, including cognitive interview protocols. One reason is to make sure certain topics or issues are explored. Thus, a section in an interview protocol will often start with a question that is entirely open-ended. Once the initial open-ended response is obtained, the interviewer follows up with probes, listed on the protocol, on possible answers the researcher wanted to explore.* For example, a researcher may be interviewing family members of those who had recently died to learn about the barriers they faced obtaining needed services. The protocol will include the initial open ended question, followed by a set of written probes such

---

*In the analysis it is critical to distinguish between statements made by the respondent without the prompting of probes and those made in response to a probe. If one wants to understand what is truly "top of mind" for a respondent, what they say at the outset has more weight.

†In a sense, such probes are responses that the researchers believe are likely to be elicited, at least from some of those interviewed. Often, however, a novice qualitative researcher will structure an interview protocol so that there is no room for the unexpected response or the response that would only be elicited from an open-ended question.

as financial barriers, lack of availability of home care services, unwillingness of physician to prescribe adequate level of pain medications, and insufficient time to care for family member and attend support groups.† Probes of this kind are quite common in even the most highly structured interviews.

Another reason for using probes is to elicit details about the respondent's "story." This is more likely in a semi-structured than a highly structured interview. For example, if the "story" is about an attempt to enroll in a low-income Medicare Savings Program, a researcher might list the following probes in questioning the target population of older people: How did they hear about the programs? How long did it take before they tried to enroll? What kind of assistance did they have? What were the barriers to enrollment they experienced? These could be conceived of as additional questions rather than as probes, but their use is to follow up on the unprompted storytelling of the respondent.

Probes are also common in cognitive interview protocols. For example, in a cognitive test of a patient education brochure that lists questions a patient might ask a doctor regarding the treatment of a particular disease, a researcher might begin by asking an open-ended question, such as, "Tell me in your own words how you would ask your doctor this question." Following this, the researcher might probe whether the person would or would not feel comfortable asking the doctor each question. The researcher might further ask whether there were terms in the written question that the person would never use and follow up by asking their reason.

The other side of the coin of structure is the extent to which the interviewer is expected to exercise autonomy and judgment. Ironically, the more autonomy the interviewer has the more the respondent is given the ability to shape the interview. An underlying value of qualitative methods, in the view of this author, is that it is based on a deep respect for the research subject, and on a desire to hear what they have to say in their own words and in a sequence that comes naturally to them.[7]

Number of Participants

While it may be natural to think of an interview as a classic dyad with one interviewer and one respondent, it is possible to have more than one interviewer and more than one respondent. Many researchers like to use two members of the research team rather than one per interview, for various reasons. The second person is not always a real "interviewer" asking questions but may be limited to taking notes (including notes on non-verbal responses if the interview is in-person) or setting up the recording equipment. Serving as an "observer" in an interview is also an excellent training opportunity for more junior members of the research team and for senior members with limited experience in qualitative work.

A second actual interviewer is typically used for important methodological reasons. Chief among these is that having a second interviewer provides the opportunity for researchers to "debrief" each other after interviews are complete. Debriefing can help, for example, if one interviewer was puzzled or uncertain about the meaning or veracity of a response to a question, or about resistance to a question. It can also help if, as is common, the answers from one respondent lead to questions or probes asked of other respondents; these important connections can emerge and be noted during the debriefing session.

How does the work get divided when there are two people asking questions? Sometimes, one person takes the lead on the entire interview, while the other inserts herself minimally, typically by asking a follow-up question. In other cases, each person can take the lead on different parts of the interview protocol; this is especially common and useful in multi-disciplinary research in which different parts of the protocol relate to different research questions. Another useful function that a second interviewer can play is to keep track of whether and when all the key questions on the protocol have been covered. This can be especially critical in a semi-structured interview where variations are made in the written question sequence.

The extent to which interviewer roles are specified ahead of time is related to the issue of structure and the history and shared experience of the two interviewers. Two people with a great deal of positive history and experience can work together seamlessly, shifting back and forth in an interview as if it were (as of course it is) a conversation.[‡]

In key informant interviews, it is also not uncommon to have multiple respondents in the same interview.[§] This can be planned, or it can happen without warning. Why would researchers plan on interviewing two or more respondents together? One circumstance is to interview couples, families, or work teams. Interviewing more than one person at a time would also make sense to obtain a narrative chronology of historical events from two or more people who share that narrative between them. For example, one might study the adoption of a new intervention within an organization, and interview people with different perspectives on the experience. Those people would be interviewed separately. But if there were two people with a highly similar perspective on the adoption experience, it might make sense to interview them together. Having each tell their part of the story as it emerged over time would shed additional light.

Why might an interviewer suddenly find himself confronted by more than one respondent? This might happen if the initial respondent felt nervous about the interview and wanted the support provided by the presence of someone of his or her own choosing. Or alternatively, the respondent might want to intimidate the interviewer with a "show of force" through numbers. It is not uncommon for a senior person to bring in a junior person because she/he thinks that person will know the answers to several of the questions (particularly questions of fact). In recent field work with area agencies on

---

[‡]This researcher has also had the joy of finding researchers with whom she could do an interview in tandem in this seamless manner literally from the outset. Shared theoretical perspectives appear to be a contributory factor.

[§]*With rare exceptions, cognitive interviews are conducted with one respondent at a time, largely because the focus is on the mental processes and personal responses of a particular individual.*

aging, the staff assumed that they would be interviewed together, not realizing that the researchers wanted to get their responses without any mediation from the presence of their supervisor, for example.

What is the difference between interviewing a group of people, especially a group of five or more, and doing a focus group? A group interview is almost always done with people who are known to each other, while a focus group is almost always done with people who are strangers. A secondary difference is that in a focus group there is a strong expectation and desire that people will react not only to the moderator's questions, but to each other's answers.[8] This dynamic is part of the "data" being acquired. In a group interview, people can and will comment on what others say. Researchers can observe the quality of their verbal (and in face to face situations, their non-verbal) interactions while simultaneously getting answers to their questions.

Mode of Administration

Qualitative interviews can be conducted by telephone or in person.[9] Mail or web-based interactions can be useful supplements to these modes, but are not effective on their own because qualitative methods depend on open-ended questions which are tedious to answer through these means. Cognitive interviews are best conducted in person, since observation of non-verbal behavior is often a critical element. It is important to keep in mind that structure and number of participants can vary in both phone and face-to-face interviews. The choice of mode of administration is one of the most critical in qualitative work; see below for a discussion of what is at stake in the choice.

Use of a Stimulus

We think of an interview in terms of a respondent answering questions. In addition, however, a stimulus can be a critical element in an interview. As described above, cognitive interviews always have a stimulus, such as a set of survey items or some kind of educational tool. Key informant interviews can also have a stimulus. A common form of stimulus is a scenario or vignette.[9,10] In one current research project, for example, the team is asking physicians to respond to vignettes about an older patient, sometimes accompanied by a younger family member, who is questioning their judgment about a hospital or specialist referral. Two vignettes are presented in turn. After each, a series of questions is asked about how the physician would respond to each vignette and why. Vignettes are used to provide a more concrete rather than an abstract frame for questions. If done well, the respondent is engaged at a deeper and, it is hoped, more realistic level. How the vignettes are crafted is of great significance. For example, these vignettes had to be provocative without being offensive. Further, they had to be realistic, both in terms of the clinical circumstances presented and the challenges made and/or the questions asked by the patient. The patient and family members also had to be drawn realistically. While vignettes and other stimuli provide structure to an interview, the interviewer can nevertheless exercise judgment in the questioning once the vignette is presented. Vignettes can be used in both in-person and telephone interviews; when the written vignette is sent ahead of time for a phone interview or handed to the respondent during an in-person interview, it can serve as a reference point during the discussion and thus make it easier for them to keep track of the material in the vignette.

Other forms of stimulus might include quantitative data or summaries of opinion on an issue. The purpose of the stimulus is to focus the respondent on specifics and avoid rambling responses that are vague and abstract.

Focus Groups

Focus groups became widely used by market researchers during the 1980s, and are still used in that context.[11] They have become a standard method for a wide range of social science research.[8] Three of the four dimensions of variation discussed above for interviews also apply to focus groups, with special twists. Since focus groups are conducted in person, there is almost no variation in mode of administration. On the other hand, the options for recording focus group interactions, such as audiotaping, videotaping, taking detailed notes, and even having a phone connection to transcribers vary considerably. In addition to how data are recorded, another important variation is whether or not the recording process is visible or invisible to the participants. This is related in turn to whether the focus group is held in a professional facility or some other setting such as an organizational meeting room or even a hotel conference center.

Almost all focus groups could be classed as semi-structured in nature. A written moderator's guide is used, parts of which are virtually a script.** The guide will typically include a number of "focus questions" and will almost always include probes. Experienced moderators like to use a guide that has "timing" noted to help them stay on track. Nevertheless, the extent and depth of responses to a question cannot always be predicted. This means that the moderator needs the autonomy to spend more time on some questions and less or no time on others, and to add probes to follow up on particularly fruitful comments or discussions.

The number of participants also varies. While there is no evidence-based answer to the question, "What's the right number?", focus groups usually consist of 5 to 15 participants. The number depends on both the length of time, the kind of participant, and the nature of the topic. Two examples help describe the range: a focus group with parents of teenage children regarding the services they need in their community included 14 people. All the participants clamored to participate and appeared eager to continue the discussion beyond the planned two hours.†† On the other hand, a set of focus groups with geriatric

---

**Scripts are particularly common at the beginning of a focus group, when the purpose, auspices and "ground rules" of the focus group discussion are presented, and when human subjects protections and informed consent are reviewed.

††*Note that this response was perhaps in itself the most telling answer to the question—these parents really wanted a chance to talk to each other!*

care managers convened to elicit their reactions to various long-term care "report cards" each included from five to eight people, lasted one hour, and elicited fruitful participation from everyone.

Although a focus group is typically moderated by one person, other members of the research team can participate either visibly or invisibly. As in interviews, "visible" participants might be managing recording equipment, taking notes privately, recording answers on newsprint for all participants to see, or handing out materials. Primarily because of its market research origins, professional focus group facilities offer the possibility of observation of the group through a two-way mirror so that the "client" can observe. In social science applications, it is more common for other members of the research team to observe, for reasons such as debriefing, training, and in many cases unobtrusive videotaping. In some cases representatives of the funder can be viewed as part of the research team. For example, senior staff at the Centers for Medicare and Medicaid Services have typically been extremely interested to observe firsthand focus groups being conducted to help refine a patient experience survey for people who have recently been hospitalized, since they play a role both in helping to articulate the policy and practice implications of the focus group research and so they can provide carefully "de-identified" summaries of the experience to their colleagues.

Focus groups are well suited for the use of one or more kinds of stimulus. Vignettes and scenarios can be used, audiotapes or videotapes can be presented, informational materials can be shared, and participants can observe or even navigate through a website. As noted above, a fairly common practice is to record the responses of focus group members as they give them. Typically, large pieces of newsprint are taped on walls around the room. Sometimes, this is done primarily to provide participants with visual confirmation of the fact that their comments have been heard. At other times, the lists are actually used as a basis for some further activity, such as clustering responses or setting priorities.

Recent technology offers the potential for immediate feedback to the group of their responses to closed-ended questions that typically tap knowledge or beliefs/opinions. The technology permits each participant to silently and privately give a response to a question by using a device resembling a remote control for a TV set. The responses are then quickly tabulated by a computer receiving the individual data, and the distribution of responses is then displayed protecting participant anonymity. These responses can then be a stimulus for further discussion. Finally, it is extremely common for focus groups to include a more closed-ended survey at some point, most commonly before the group itself begins. These surveys typically include questions about participants that go beyond what was collected during the screening process, as well as questions on participants' knowledge, attitudes, beliefs, opinions, and experiences prior to participation in the group. In some cases, researchers may conceive of the focus group as both a data collection method as well as an "intervention." In such situations, surveys may actually be re-administered at the end.

Observation

Observation is a somewhat neglected data collection method, whether used on its own or as an element of in-person interviews and focus groups, which always provide opportunities to observe as well as to ask questions.[1] While the word "observation" seems to imply "looking," an observation can involve other senses such as hearing, smelling, and awareness of climate in its original rather than metaphorical use.

The value of observation is that researchers are one step closer to empirical reality. They not asking someone what happened, but they are seeing, listening to, and directly experiencing what happened. In qualitative "question asking," researchers must always be aware that the respondents are filtering what they have experienced and reporting only some of it, based on their particular perspective. When observing, the researchers have to transfer that awareness to themselves. Respondents are filtering; researchers are observing and reporting from their own perspective. While this does not make the observation invalid, it requires, as in all qualitative methods, a rigorous approach that leaves great opportunity for the researcher to learn if any presuppositions are incorrect and any emergent hypotheses are wrong-headed.

What can be observed? The list is endless and includes meetings, the process of seeking and receiving services, training and educational sessions, policy-related events such as hearings, debates, news conferences, or interviews; and, an especially underutilized approach, the details of a physical setting or environment. For the most part, what is observed is behavior, interactions or settings, or most typically a combination of all three. Settings are especially under-observed, even though they can be powerful shapers of behavior and interactions, as well as reflecting values and assumptions. For example, if the researcher enters a service delivery site, she/he might want to observe the population density of the staff; the extent of disparity in the size, the privacy, and the quality of office space reflecting organizational hierarchy; the size and comfort of the waiting rooms; the degree of privacy afforded to staff–client interactions; aspects of the environment such as temperature, noise level and source(s) of noise; how new the furniture looks; how messy the desks are; or whether there is both "organizationally" and "personally" chosen art works, plants, and the like.

A major variation in observation is between direct, indirect, and participant observation. In direct observation the researcher is simply an observer. In indirect observation technology is used to capture something the researcher wants to observe without the presence of the researcher.‡‡ In participant observation the researchers are participating actively in whatever they are observing.[12]

Another major variation in observation is the extent of structure. Participant observation is almost always fairly unstructured, while both direct and indirect observation can range from unstructured to highly structured. In the context of observation, structure means deliberately focusing on certain

---

‡‡It could be argued that indirect observation is highly akin to, perhaps indistinguishable from, the collection of texts and images for analysis.

dimensions of what is being observed. If a researcher goes to a meeting of twenty people, what does she/he watch? What does she/he listen for? The possibilities are almost infinite. However, if the researcher has a research question, then as in all good inquiry, that question should drive the data collection decisions. In qualitative work, there is always the desire to stay open and responsive, and that is true in even the most highly structured observation. One needs, both literally and metaphorically, to have good peripheral vision, even though in a structured or semi-structured observation the researcher enters the situation with a fairly clear idea of how to direct his or her eyes, ears, and other senses.

The way to build structure into observations is to construct an observation protocol, which is often in the form of a series of questions. Typically, the questions in an observation protocol will reflect not only the research questions, but the theoretical or conceptual roots of the study. For example, a protocol for observing a staff or team meeting is likely to derive primarily from theories and research in management and group dynamics. Implicit in the questions are hypotheses about the features of a group interaction that predict the effectiveness of a group in both completing tasks and supporting group cohesion and development. Constructing an observation protocol offers an opportunity to surface the researcher's hypotheses and assumptions.

Another advantage of using a protocol is that if the questions are descriptive, as they should be, the researcher will focus on and record exactly what was seen/heard/felt, and postpone until later interpreting what happened. The "raw data," i.e., the observation notes, can then be reviewed by others to identify alternative interpretations. This does not mean that the observer is prohibited from noting down interpretations, however. Interpretations should be labeled as such so that they can be considered and reconsidered.

What is at Stake in Data Collection Decisions?

Basic choices about data collection methods are driven by the nature of the research question and by the nature of the researcher's unit of analysis (organization, family, team, individual, community, patient-physician dyad, etc.). These factors inform what kind of data, from whom or where, will be most relevant.

In any study there are several data collection choices. The choices should take into consideration other important factors, including 1) the quality of the data, including its completeness, depth, and credibility, in particular; 2) the time and costs to collect the data; and 3) the opportunities to build capacity for the future.

The methods a researcher chooses influence several aspects of data quality, including whether one can: 1) collect data from the right respondents or about the right events; 2) question enough respondents or observe enough events; 3) create a context that helps respondents be honest, accurate, and engaged[§§];

[§§]One advantage of observations is that one is most often going to the settings of research subjects in which they live and work.

4) get the desired depth and breadth of information; 5) have the data collected by people with the most appropriate skills; and 6) acquire the information in a form easily amenable to data management and analysis. The time and cost of data collection is related not only to the broad choice of method but to the more specific choices within each method. Data collection choices, finally, determine whether or not a researcher can provide opportunities to build the capacity of those new to qualitative methods.

An example will illustrate how consideration of these issues can influence decisions, both individually and collectively. We conducted a formative evaluation of a rotation in the second year of an internal medicine residency program. During the rotation, residents accompanied physician faculty as they made home visits as part of a highly structured service to primarily elderly, home-bound patients with complex medical conditions. The purpose of the study was to describe the nature of this educational intervention and acquire a preliminary understanding of potential outcomes for the medical residents. The research team had three members, all of whom were experienced in interviews; two of the three were less experienced in observations.

We used key informant interviews of a wide range of program participants. We also conducted protocol-driven observations of various seminars and meetings that the residents attended during the month rotation. We did *not* observe the actual home visits, primarily because we did not want to intrude into the patients' homes in case this could make them uncomfortable. Though we paid a high price for this choice, we continue to think it was the ethically sound decision, given the level of frailty and frequent cognitive impairment of the patients and the fact that they were already dealing with a newcomer in the form of the resident.

We also did *not* conduct focus groups with the residents. We conducted our research during approximately six rotations. The three or four residents in each cycle were too few for an effective focus group. Further, since the residents knew each other well, it would have been more like a group interview than a focus group. But we rejected group interviews as well as conducting a focus group with residents from multiple rotations. In our judgment, it would be superior to conduct an individual in-person interview with each resident at the outset and the end of the rotation. In an individual interview we could collect in-depth data on many issues. We also reasoned that if no other residents were present, individuals would be less subject to filtering what they said based on social desirability criteria. An in-person interview would, we thought, also be more likely to support rapport between interviewer and respondent and reduce respondent uncertainty about who we were and why we were doing this study. In-person interviews, at the home base of the respondents where they would be most comfortable, were also feasible since the program setting was in our city.

Accordingly, we developed a semi-structured protocol, with lots of probes. Had our interview team included less experienced researchers, we might have used a more structured protocol. Even given experienced researchers, however, an entirely unstructured approach would have made it difficult to aggregate findings across interviews, particularly those with residents. As it was, interviewers had considerable autonomy in question wording and sequencing. We used only one researcher in interviews with residents, both to avoid "outnumbering" the respondent and to maximize the number of interviews we could conduct. This was a difficult decision since it meant sacrificing the potential benefit of having interviewers debrief after each interview. However, since interviews were tape-recorded and transcribed, the results were available for review by all three members of the research team. Avoiding complexity in scheduling was a logistical issue that supported the use of a single interviewer. Two of the three members of the research team had multiple other responsibilities, making it difficult to schedule two to one, as compared to one to one interviews.

We also conducted semi-structured interviews with all the clinicians associated with the program, with senior leaders in both the medical school and the affiliated medical center, and with staff of home health agencies with whom the program worked. Two researchers participated in about a quarter of these interviews, especially those with organizational leaders. We were not worried that these informants would be less forthcoming if more than one person were present because they had considerable organizational standing and influence and would be less likely to be intimidated by a researcher doing an interview. More interviews were done with a pair of interviewers early in the project, to provide an opportunity for the least senior member of the research team to observe the interviewing "style" of the other members. However, the two most experienced members also did interviews together, especially with high level organizational leaders, both because we wanted the opportunity to debrief afterwards, and because we so enjoyed interviewing together.

What about our observations? In each rotation, there were several kinds of educational interactions we observed, including the initial orientation meeting and four distinct weekly seminars. Observation protocols were used for all these events. Only one member of the research team was present in these direct observations. This person was visible but worked to be unobtrusive and to avoid verbal comments and visible non-verbal reactions. Over the course of a given rotation, it proved easy for everyone to ignore us, even when we chose to take notes on a laptop computer rather than by hand. Although only one observer was present at a time, the multiplicity of rotations we observed made it possible for each member of the team to observe each type of event at least once. Wherever possible, we observed the entire "sequence" of a seminar, rather than only one or two sessions, to make sure we could observe how the dynamics of the residents with each other and with the faculty developed and changed over time, among other things. Having a team of three members and the proximity of the site made this feasible.

A Methodological Research Agenda

As the use of qualitative methods increases, it becomes more important to systematically learn about the consequences of data collection choices. Here are some research questions that could benefit from methodological studies:
1) What is the impact of degree of structure in interviews with elites? With patients or otherwise vulnerable populations? Under which circumstances

is more detail obtained? What is the nature and extent of inconsistencies in the actual content of responses in interviews with varying levels of structure?

2) Similarly, what is the impact of mode of administration in interviews? What kind of non-verbal responses can actually be collected during in-person interviews that add value to the information that can be obtained by phone? What in particular is the affect of mode of administration on the extent and content of responses to "sensitive" questions?

3) What do research subjects across data collection methods report, after the fact, about their level of comfort during data collection? For example, did they think privacy was invaded? Were they asked questions that were difficult or distressing to answer? Did they share all the information they could have and, if not, why did they hold back information? Did they share everything they wanted to and, if not, what stopped them? Did their behavior change when they were being observed, and if so, how? How did they respond to such variations as multiple interviewers, visible or non-visible recording, or the size of a focus group?

4) What benefits, if any, do research subjects across methods report as arising from their participation?

Answers to these questions can help both researchers and their audiences have more confidence in the appropriateness of their data collection decisions. Such studies will not eliminate the need for judgment to be exercised, but they can both heighten and deepen our awareness of how subtle variations can influence the quality, indeed the nature, of the data we collect.

This chapter has presented the range of methods available within the tradition of qualitative research, including interviews, focus groups, and observation. We have explored within each of these major methods how specific data collection efforts are shaped through decisions made about how much structure should be imposed on data collection; how many people are involved on both sides of the data collection "table"; whether data are collected in person or by phone; and whether a stimulus is used to aid in data collection. We have used examples from our own research experience to illustrate how the myriad decisions made in collecting qualitative data are driven by the nature of the research question, the experience of the research team, the characteristics of research subjects, and of course by what is feasible. Attention to these details can have a substantial impact on whether qualitative research results in meaningful findings that generate confidence.

Summary Points

- A wide range of data collection methods is available for use within qualitative research traditions, including key informant and cognitive interviews, focus groups, and observation.
- Decisions about data collection methods are driven by the nature of the research question and the proposed unit of analysis (organization, family, team, individual, community, patient-physician dyad, etc.).
- Choice of data collection method influences data quality in several ways, including the relevance of data gathered, availability of sufficient respondents or events, candor and honesty of respondents, the desired depth and breadth of information, appropriateness of data collector skills, and suitability of the data for analysis.
- There are four major dimensions of variation in the design of interviews: the degree of structure, the number of participants, the mode of administration, and the nature of the stimulus to generate responses.

References

1) Patton, M.Q. *Qualitative Research and Evaluation Methods*. 3rd ed. Thousand Oaks, CA: Sage Publications; 2002.
2) Rubin H.J. and Rubin, I.S. *Qualitative Interviewing*. 2nd ed. Thousand Oaks, CA: Sage Publications; 2004.
3) DeMaio, T.J. and Rothbeg, J.M. Cognitive Interviewing Techniques in the Lab and in the Field. In: Schwartz, N. and Sudman, S., eds. *Answering Questions: Methodology for Determining Cognitive and Communicative Processes in Survey Research*. San Francisco: Jossey-Bass; 1996:177.
4) Willis, G.B. *Cognitive Interviewing: A Tool for Improving Questionnaire Design*. Thousand Oaks, CA: Sage Publications; 2004.
5) McGee, J., Kanouse, D.E., Sofaer, S., Hargraves, L., Kleimann, S., and Hoy, E.W. Making Survey Results Easy to Report to Consumers: How Reporting Needs Guided Survey Development in CAHPS. *Med Care*. 1999; 37:MS32-MS40.
6) Briggs, C.L. Questions for the Ethnographer: A Critical Examination of the Role of the Interview in Fieldwork. In: Bryman, A., ed. *Ethnography, Volume 2: Ethnographic Fieldwork Practice* Thousand Oaks, CA: Sage Publications; 2001.
7) Sofaer, S. Qualitative Research Methods: What are They and why use Them? *Health Services Research*. 1999; 34: 1101-1118.
8) Morgan, D.L. *Focus Groups as Qualitative Research* 1996. Thousand Oaks, CA: Sage Publications; Patton MQ. *Qualitative Research and Evaluation Methods*. 3rd ed. Thousand Oaks, CA: Sage Publications; 2001.
9) Shuy, R.W. In Person Versus Telephone Interviewing. In: Holstein, J. and Gubrium, J., eds. *Inside Interviewing: New Lenses, New Concerns*. Thousand Oaks, CA: Sage Publications; 2003.
10) Barter, C. and Renold, E. I Wanna Tell You a Story: Exploring the Application of Vignettes in Qualitative Research with Children and Young People. *International Journal of Social Research Methodology*. 2000; 3:307-324.
11) Mariampolski, H. *Qualitative Market Research*. Thousand Oaks, CA: Sage Publications; 2001.
12) Platt, J. The Development of the "Participant Observation" Method in Sociology. In: Bryman, A., ed. *Ethnography, Volume 1: The Nature of Ethnography* Thousand Oaks, CA: Sage Publications; 2001.

Chapter 5

"Connected Contributions" as a Motivation for Combining Qualitative and Quantitative Methods

David L. Morgan, PhD

Introduction

This chapter provides practical advice about how to integrate qualitative and quantitative methods. It assumes that you have already made decisions about the kinds of knowledge you want to produce, and that you are ready to pursue a research design. This practical orientation does not mean, however, that this chapter will be a "how-to manual." In particular, the first step in deciding how to combine qualitative and quantitative methods is to understand why you want to use multiple methods.

There is universal recognition that different methods have different strengths, and the desire to take advantage of these different strengths provides the basic motivation for combining methods. Unfortunately, this motivation is too vague to provide much guidance in selecting an actual research design. In addition, concentrating solely on the benefits of combining different strengths of multiple methods ignores the complexity involved in projects that bring together the very different tools and traditions involved in qualitative and quantitative research. Ultimately, you will need to integrate what you learn from each of the methods that you use—a task that can be extremely challenging if you do not begin with a carefully developed and strong research design. One way to move beyond the broad justification offered by an emphasis on "different strengths" is to match your own purposes to the goals that have motivated other researchers in their efforts to combine qualitative and quantitative methods.

Combining Methods

Triangulation

Three broad motivations have provided the basis for most applications of multiple methods. The oldest and best-known of these motivations is triangulation, which involves using two different methods to study the same question, and then assessing the extent to which they agree.[1,2] Here, your goal is to demonstrate that methods with very different strengths produce findings that "converge" like the tip of a triangle. For example, if you were investigating how a new policy affects a particular group, you could compare statistical data on those changes with open-ended interviews from those experiencing the changes. Despite its long history, triangulation is not currently a common motivation for combining methods, partly because it is often inefficient to devote considerable resources to the limited goal of "answering the same question twice," and partly because this approach does not address the all-too-common problem of what to do when your methods yield different results.

Expanded Coverage

A second motivation for using multiple methods is to assign each method a separate purpose, so that the combination provides expanded coverage of your research topic. Denzin[2] and others[3] originally proposed expanded coverage as an alternative to triangulation, based on a division of labor where different methods serve different goals, depending on their specific strengths. This approach addresses the inefficiency of using multiple methods to answer the same question, while also eliminating concerns about the extent to which the methods disagree. For example, a survey that provided broad descriptive data about a population could be combined with a series of case studies that provided more depth and detail about a specific set of sites. Unfortunately, expanded coverage has yet to develop into a well-defined set of research designs. One difficulty is that a narrow emphasis on expanded coverage can create as many problems as it solves, primarily because it fails to address the issue of integration. In particular, it is rare to find such a total division of labor that you can use the qualitative and quantitative methods for completely separate purposes; instead, there are likely to be areas of overlap, so you still must face the question of how to compare and integrate the different kinds of results that these methods produce.

Connected Contributions

The third motivation for combining methods applies what you learn from one method to enhance your ability to use another method through connected contributions.[4,5] In this approach, you also follow the logic of assigning methods to different goals within the overall study, while confronting the question of integration by using the results from one method to enhance the performance of another method. Rather than the complete separation that is often implied in expanded coverage, research motivated by connected contributions explicitly links the designs for the different methods. For example, an exploratory qualitative study might be followed by a quantitative study that was designed to test the insights gained from that earlier research. Like the previous two motivations, connected contributions often has the problem that what sounds good in principle can be difficult to put into practice. The bulk of this chapter will describe a set of practical research designs that integrate the different strengths of qualitative and quantitative methods through connected contributions.

Connected contributions has several practical advantages over both triangulation and expanded coverage. On the one hand, triangulation offers a well-developed approach that suffers from a limited set of purposes and raises questions about what to do in the face of conflicting results. On the other hand, expanded coverage has not provided a basis for clear-cut research designs, and also suffers from some of the same problems as triangulation. Connected contributions currently offers the best alternative for creating a series of research designs that will allow practicing researchers to pursue a well-defined set of motivations for combining multiple methods.

The next section describes four research designs that use sequential priorities as a strategy for implementing connected contributions. As Figure 1 shows, each of these designs combines a qualitative and a quantitative method, based on two options for the sequence in which you use these methods and two options for the priority that you assign to each method.

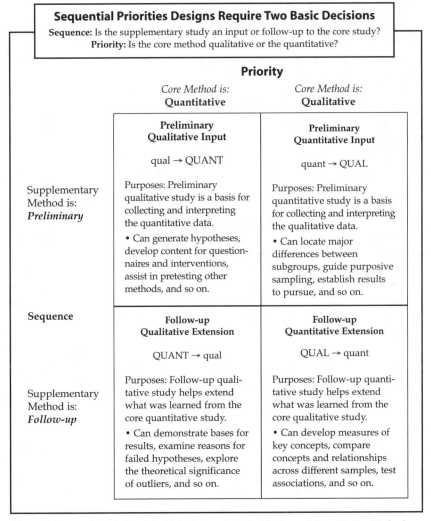

Sequential Priorities Designs Require Two Basic Decisions

Sequence: Is the supplementary study an input or follow-up to the core study?
Priority: Is the core method qualitative or the quantitative?

	Priority	
	Core Method is: **Quantitative**	*Core Method is:* **Qualitative**
Supplementary Method is: *Preliminary*	**Preliminary Qualitative Input** qual → QUANT Purposes: Preliminary qualitative study is a basis for collecting and interpreting the quantitative data. • Can generate hypotheses, develop content for questionnaires and interventions, assist in pretesting other methods, and so on.	**Preliminary Quantitative Input** quant → QUAL Purposes: Preliminary quantitative study is a basis for collecting and interpreting the qualitative data. • Can locate major differences between subgroups, guide purposive sampling, establish results to pursue, and so on.
Sequence **Supplementary Method is:** *Follow-up*	**Follow-up Qualitative Extension** QUANT → qual Purposes: Follow-up qualitative study helps extend what was learned from the core quantitative study. • Can demonstrate bases for results, examine reasons for failed hypotheses, explore the theoretical significance of outliers, and so on.	**Follow-up Quantitative Extension** QUAL → quant Purposes: Follow-up quantitative study helps extend what was learned from the core qualitative study. • Can develop measures of key concepts, compare concepts and relationships across different samples, test associations, and so on.

Figure 1. Sequential Priorities Model for Integrating Qualitative and Quantitative Methods

Preliminary Qualitative Input

In preliminary qualitative input designs, the first stage of the project is a supplementary qualitative study that contributes to the development of the core, quantitative portion of the project. This design uses the strength of qualitative input to enhance the effectiveness of either a quantitative survey or an experimental program intervention. Both of these quantitative methods require predetermined data collection procedures, which remain "fixed" after they are put into use. Preliminary qualitative studies are especially useful for developing the content of surveys and intervention programs, by providing insight into the issues that matter most to the research participants themselves.

For surveys, the key use of a preliminary qualitative input design is to help develop the questionnaire itself. If you are working in a new area, where you have limited experience investigating a topic or a category of respondents, qualitative methods can help you discover the issues that matter most and the language respondents use to discuss these issues. Whenever you are uncertain about which topics you need to include in your questions, exploratory qualitative methods can help you determine the domains that you need to cover. In other cases, the broad interview topics will be set and the qualitative methods will help you understand the participants' perspectives on these topics. For example, even when there are existing survey instruments in an area of study, you may want to be sure that those items convey the desired meaning for the people you will be interviewing— especially when you are working with a new research population. In addition to locating either the topics that should be included in the interview or the types of questions that can tap into those topics, qualitative methods are also useful for assessing the wording of the items you intend to use. For example, most forms of "cognitive interviewing"[6] use variations on qualitative methods to determine not only whether the respondents correctly interpret the meaning of the questions, but also whether the questions have the same meaning to different groups of respondents (e.g., younger and older respondents or blacks and whites).

For program interventions, preliminary qualitative input designs can help in selecting the actual target for the intervention and in refining the design of the intervention, as well as assisting in both the measurement of key concepts and the implementation of more specific aspects of the program. With regard to determining the behaviors targeted for the intervention, this approach is especially valuable when you are relatively unfamiliar with either the behaviors you want to change or the people who will be participating in the program. For example, when you are extending your work to include new cultural groups, qualitative methods can help you understand the research participants' basic needs and their feelings about different forms of service delivery that could meet those needs. With regard to the measurement of key concepts, qualitative methods can help identify which types of outcomes to measure and how best to capture those results. In addition, qualitative methods can often point to a wider range of program impacts and generate additional outcome measures that may be more sensitive to the experiences and preferences of the program participants. With regard to implementing specific aspects of the program, qualitative methods can help you understand the participants' perspective, including the various factors that will affect their participation. For example, participant observation in a similar service setting or open-ended interviewing with potential clients can provide insight into the kind of access and convenience issues that often have a major impact on the extent to which services are used. It does researchers little good to design an excellent set of services if the target population believes that it is difficult to use those services.

Among the four specific designs considered here, preliminary qualitative input designs have received the most explicit attention in the methodological literature. In part, this is due to the fact that these designs reflect the dominant or core position of quantitative methods in many fields. This reason does not, however, diminish the strengths that qualitative methods can offer as preliminary input to quantitative methods, along with the desirability of any input that can strengthen the quality of a survey instrument or a program intervention. One recent recognition of the value of this kind of research is the National Institutes of Health's establishment of awards for "Exploratory-Developmental Research" (R-21), which are, according to the NIH website "intended to encourage new, exploratory, and developmental research projects by providing support for the early stages of their development." (Note, however, that some NIH Institutes and Centers do not currently accept R-21 applications.)

Preliminary Quantitative Input

For preliminary quantitative input designs, the first stage of the project is a supplementary quantitative study that contributes to the development of the core, qualitative portion of the project. This design uses the strengths of quantitative methods as inputs to enhance the effectiveness of either open-ended interviewing or participant observation. Both of these qualitative methods can benefit from systematic procedures for selecting data sources through "purposive" or "theoretical" sampling,[8] rather than relying on "convenience samples." Given the small number of data sources in most studies that use open-ended interviewing or participant observation, it is especially important to select the "right" cases. Preliminary quantitative input designs can contribute to the effectiveness of qualitative studies by providing a systematic, purposive approach for selecting data sources by locating cases through existing databases.

Open-ended interviewing can benefit from preliminary quantitative input studies that help locate research participants who can serve as rich sources of information about the specific purposes of the research. The sources for this quantitative data range from surveys that point to specific individuals, to impersonal sources of aggregate data that help in locating particular categories of informants. Using an existing survey as the source to recruit your research participants can create the opportunity to contact specific types of individuals who would be difficult to find in other ways. By using the variables from a survey to do systematic screening and determine eligibility, you can locate interview informants who meet very specific selection criteria. Organizational databases can also serve as useful screening devices to locate participants in purposively determined categories, and this strategy is especially useful for comparative purposes. For example, you might want to select your respondents according to criteria such as age, gender, years of residence, geographical location, and so on. Even impersonal, aggregate data sources such as censuses, maps, and government documents can provide a useful tool for locating broad categories of research participants. For example, these sources could help you locate people in areas according to income levels, housing values, family composition, and the relative availability of a variety of services.

Participant observation and other types of "case studies" can be even more sensitive to the selection of data sources, since these methods often rely on only a single site or at most several. Given the importance of selecting appropriate locations for case studies, it would be surprising not to use sources such as censuses, maps, and government documents—both to help in the selection of study sites and to provide important contextual information about those sites. Organizational databases can also play an important role in the selection of cases, and this type of quantitative data is once again particularly useful in comparative research. For example, although it would be inappropriate to generalize from a handful of "randomly selected" cases in an organizational database, it would be much more effective to use those records to compare sets of cases that differ according to some theoretically important selection factor. Finally, when you have survey data that were collected at the organizational level, there is the potential for selecting cases according to very detailed eligibility criteria. For example, if you are looking for a site with unusual characteristics, a systematic search through survey data may help you locate just such an "outlier."

Although preliminary quantitative input designs have not received as much explicit attention as projects that begin with preliminary qualitative studies, there is little doubt that this approach is a common strategy in qualitative research. The current goal is thus to call attention to the advantages that preliminary quantitative input designs offer the researcher, and to urge more direct effort in explicitly developing this design. Funded research is one area where preliminary quantitative input may be especially valuable for largely qualitative projects, by addressing concerns that the sources for the data will be selected in some haphazard or "biased" way. While the purpose of qualitative research is seldom to generalize to larger populations, it is still important to use systematic and carefully chosen criteria in selecting data sources, and preliminary quantitative input designs offer clear strengths in this regard.

Follow-Up Qualitative Extension

For follow-up qualitative extension designs, the first stage of the project is the core, quantitative method, followed by a supplementary qualitative study that expands on what was learned in the quantitative portion of the study. This design uses the strengths that qualitative methods provide to improve on what has been learned through either a survey or an experimental program intervention. The follow-up qualitative extension provides the researcher the opportunity to move beyond the limitations of simply analyzing the quantitative data, which in itself may not be enough to help you fully understand analytic results. Follow-up qualitative studies allow you to go beyond the data you already have by exploring the experiences and circumstances that influenced and produced the initial quantitative data set.

When survey research produces unexpected results, it may be difficult to explore or interpret those results without collecting new data, and this is an excellent use for follow-up qualitative extension designs. The most obvious situation where this occurs is with results that come out "significant in the wrong direction," that is, statistically significant in the opposite direction of the original hypothesis. While the original data may provide some resources for investigating this situation, the fact that you were wrong in your original predictions suggests that you might do well to talk to the respondents who actually produced the results, rather than rely on your own judgment. There can also be benefits for pursuing cases where the results are merely "non-significant" rather than significant in either direction. In particular, if the non-significant results are associated with a central prediction in the study, it may be worth investigating why the central hypothesis was not supported. Even in analyses that do match your original predications, there may be additional interesting information to be obtained by paying attention to outliers. In this case, you are not looking for interesting cases that can serve as the basis for a full-scale qualitative study; instead, your goal is to increase your overall understanding by examining unusual cases that fall outside the normal pattern. For example, it is common to find that higher levels of resources lead to better outcomes, but you might also want to examine cases in which low resources somehow still produced good outcomes or cases where high resource levels were associated with relatively poor outcomes.

Follow-up qualitative extension designs can also be useful for understanding the results of intervention programs. All too often, the results from an experimental intervention are only "marginally significant," producing a relatively wide distribution of outcomes rather than across-the-board benefits. When your results fit that pattern, it makes sense to pursue exploratory research that searches for systematic differences between the high- and low-performing cases in the dataset. One possible outcome from this kind of study is more selective targeting of the intervention in future uses. In this circumstance, the exploratory research generates hypotheses about the factors that make the intervention more likely to work in some situations and less likely in others, so that future interventions can be more effectively targeted to the cases where the program has the best chance of being effective. Another possible outcome emphasizes tailoring the future applications of the program. In that instance, you would generate hypotheses about factors that are either facilitators for or barriers to success, so that different versions of the program could be tailored to various sites, according to the profile of facilitators and barriers at a given location.

Follow-up qualitative extension designs are currently not as well known as either of the two designs based on preliminary inputs, but interest in these designs is increasing. One possible reason for this increased interest is the current dilemma that quantitative researchers encounter in the face of weak results—currently, if you can't reject the null hypothesis, all too often your only other choice is to throw away the data. Yet, because those data were often based on strong theory and well-developed methods, it would be highly desirable to understand the sources of the results. Furthermore, with program interventions, it would be wasteful to abandon the substantial investment that often goes into that work, when a more carefully targeted or tailored version of the intervention might prove more effective. Interestingly, it can be difficult to obtain external funding for follow-up qualitative extension, because the suggestion that you might want to explore the results of your quantitative methods implies that your research design may not work as promised. This lack of support for exploratory follow-up research is especially ironic because it limits the options for understanding unsuccessful projects that even the experts on the review committee rated as likely to succeed. One way to address this problem is to begin with a plan to study outliers from your predicted results, since it is always worthwhile to extend our understanding of a successful set of results; then, if the results do not turn out as planned, you ask to reallocate those resources accordingly. Another option would be to apply for an additional study as part of your "continuing" work—possibly using something like NIH's Exploratory/Developmental (R-21) mechanism. Either way, there is a great deal to be said for gaining a better understanding of the results from your research, and this is especially true when a project produces unexpected results.

Follow-Up Quantitative Extension

For follow-up quantitative extension designs, the first stage of the project is the core, qualitative method, followed by a supplementary quantitative study that expands on what you accomplish in the qualitative portion of the study. This design uses the strengths of quantitative methods in a follow-up study that adds to the effectiveness of either open-ended interviewing or participant observation. Both of these qualitative methods typically involve small numbers of cases in which the investigator was highly involved in collecting and interpreting the data, which can limit the extent to which your conclusions are transferable to other cases. Follow-up quantitative studies allow you to go beyond the data you already have to examine whether you can demonstrate similar results for other people or settings.

When the core, qualitative study is based on open-ended interviewing, one of the most effective uses for a follow-up quantitative extension is to show that your results apply to a wider range of people than just the relatively small number of informants who typically participate in a qualitative study. Survey research is particularly useful for this purpose, and these kinds of supplementary, follow-up surveys may be relatively simple. In particular, with regard to the survey instrument itself, the fact that you are not going to engage in elaborate statistical analyses means that your questions can rely on "face validity"—that is, a general agreement that they measure what you intend to measure. Similarly, with regard to sampling, you are unlikely to need representative estimates of the scores in a larger population, because your goal is simply to show that your conclusions apply to more people than just the ones in your original study. In other words, your goal in this kind of design is not to do a full-scale piece of quantitative research, but rather to use some of the strengths of qualitative methods in a carefully focused strategy in order to support a claim that your results are more widespread.

A similar logic applies when the core, qualitative study is based on participant observation, and you want to claim that your results can be applied in settings beyond the ones you observed—what qualitative researchers refer to as the transferability of your results.[9] In that case, your follow-up quantitative extension study might take the form of a small "demonstration program," to test the extent to which your insights from an initial set of cases can produce similar results in other settings. Here, your goal is to show that the conclusions you reached in one setting point to an intervention that will produce a desired outcome in another, related setting. This kind of demonstration program typically does not require all the complexity of a full-scale intervention, because your goal is essentially to generate a "proof of concept" and not to make larger claims about the magnitude of the effects that your program might produce. Once again, this kind of supplementary follow-up study often does not need to be as extensive as a true, stand-alone quantitative study would be.

If you want to demonstrate that the results from open-ended interviewing apply to a wider range of people or that the processes you observed in case studies can be transferred to other settings, then follow-up quantitative extension designs are well suited to these purposes. Note, however, that this statement is quite different from saying that qualitative research is not "complete" or "proven" until it has been tested with quantitative methods. Instead, follow-up quantitative extension designs are intended specifically for situations where you want to extend the results from your original qualitative study. Many qualitative studies are complete and stand on their own without any quantitative follow-ups. When your goals include making claims about the generality or the transferability of your results, however, it would usually be quite inefficient to continue with in-depth interviews or case studies. This is where the strengths of follow-up quantitative extension designs are most relevant.

Conclusions

These four research designs are by no means the only ways to integrate qualitative and quantitative methods. Instead, they represent one set of practical alternatives, which address many of the reasons why social science researchers want to combine methods. Ultimately, any approach to research design has two goals: to show you the options that are available, and to provide guidance about how to choose among those options. This chapter introduces the concept of "Connected Contributions" and provides a rationale for this approach to integrating qualitative and quantitative methods.

Summary Points
- Motivations for using mixed methods include triangulation, expanded coverage and "connected contributions" (when findings from one method enhance your ability to use another method).
- Preliminary qualitative input designs use a supplementary qualitative study that contributes to the development of the core, quantitative portion of the project, enhancing the effectiveness of either a quantitative survey or an experimental program intervention.
- Preliminary quantitative input designs use a supplementary quantitative study that contributes to the development of the core, qualitative portion of the project, enhancing the effectiveness of either open-ended interviewing or participant observation.
- Follow-up qualitative extension designs have a core, quantitative method, followed by a supplementary qualitative study that expands on what was learned in the quantitative portion of the study.
- Follow-up quantitative extension designs have a core, qualitative method, followed by a supplementary quantitative study that expands on what was accomplished in the qualitative portion of the study.

References

1) Webb, E.J., Campbell, D.T., et al. *Unobtrusive Measures: Nonreactive Research in the Social Sciences* (2nd Edition). Boston: Houghton Mifflin, 1988.
2) Denzin, N.K. *The Research Act: A Theoretical Introduction to Sociological Methods* (3rd Edition). Englewood Cliffs, NJ: Prentice Hall, 1989.
3) Fielding, N. and Fielding, J.L. *Linking Data*. Thousand Oaks, CA: Sage Publications, 1986.
4) Morgan, D.L. Practical Strategies for Combining Qualitative and Quantitative Methods: Applications to Health Research. *Qualitative Health Research*. 1998; 8: 362-376.
5) Morgan, D.L. *Integrating Qualitative and Quantitative Methods*. Thousand Oaks, CA: Sage Publications, 2006.
6) Krause, N., Chatters, L.M., Meltzer, T., and Morgan, D.L. Using Focus Groups to Explore the Nature of Prayer in Late Life. *Journal of Aging Studies*. 2000; 14: 191-212.

7) Presser, S., Rothgeb, J.M., et al. *Methods for Testing and Evaluating Survey Questionnaires*. Hoboken, NJ: Wiley Interscience, 2004.

8) Patton, M.Q., *Qualitative Research and Evaluation Methods* (3rd edition). Thousand Oaks, CA: Sage Publications, 2002.

9) Lincoln, Y.S. and Guba, E.G. *Naturalistic Inquiry*. Thousand Oaks, CA: Sage Publications, 1985.

Chapter 6

Principles and Procedures of Maintaining Validity for Mixed-Method Design

Janice M. Morse, PhD (Nurs), PhD (Anthro), D.Nurs.,
Ruth R. Wolfe, MPH, and Linda Niehaus, PhD

Introduction

The exploratory nature of research, the complexities of the phenomena being studied, and the limitations within methods mean that there are occasions when a phenomenon cannot be described in its entirety using a single method. Sometimes, to comprehensively address the research question, a project using both qualitative and quantitative methods must be proposed. At other times, unexpected findings emerge that demand to be addressed during the course of a project. Sometimes these findings may best be addressed using another methodological strategy. For instance, in a qualitatively-driven project a need for *measurement* of certain aspects of the phenomenon may arise, demanding the use of a quantitative strategy. Similarly, during a quantitatively-driven project, surprising findings that occur during the analysis may indicate the need for additional description using a qualitative strategy. Such possibilities mean that, in order to complete the study, a mixed-method design must be used. This approach would incorporate a supplementary component that may or may not have been anticipated at the proposal stage.* The purpose of this chapter is to review the principles of mixed-method design and to explicate the procedures that are required to permit strategies from apparently incompatible paradigms to coexist within the same project without threatening validity.

Mixed-method research is a design which encompasses several variations: one in which the core component of the research is qualitative, with a supplementary quantitative component (QUAL ±> quan); another with a supplementary qualitative component (QUAL ±> qual) (*see* Box 1). Alternatively, it may have a quantitative core component, with a supplementary qualitative component (QUAN ±> qual)[1] or another quantitative component (QUAN ±> quan). Nomenclature for different types of mixed-method designs is presented in Box 1. CAPS are used to denote the core component of the

---

*Adopting supplementary strategies in the course of a research project may have other practical implications, such as requiring additional ethics review, extending timelines, additional funding, additional expertise, and so on, and these technical aspects of conducting research must be attended to by the researcher.

project while the supplementary component of the project is indicated in lower case. Also of importance is the pacing of the supplementary component. If this component is conducted at the same time as the core component of the project, the design is then *simultaneous*, indicated with a + sign; if the supplementary component follows the core component, it is *sequential*, and indicated with a -> sign. In this chapter we only address (QUAL ±> quan) and (QUAN ±> qual) mixed-method designs because these designs have the greatest potential for error and threats to validity. Further clarification about these issues is provided below.

"Mixed-method design" introduces new terminology, and these terms are listed in Box 2 . The *core* component of the project is the primary or main study, and the *supplementary* component consists of strategies added to obtain desired supplemental information. In mixed-method design, the core component is complete (i.e., scientifically rigorous) and can therefore stand alone, while the supplemental component is conducted only to the extent that the researcher is certain the findings are adequate to provide the necessary additional information to address the research question. We therefore refer to the research

Box 1: Nomenclature for types of Mixed-Method Design

QUAL + quan:	Qualitative core component of the project (inductive theoretical drive) with a simultaneous quantitative supplementary component.
QUAL -> quan:	Qualitative core component of the project (inductive theoretical drive) with a sequential quantitative supplementary component.
QUAL + qual:	Qualitative core component of the project (inductive theoretical drive) with a simultaneous qualitative supplementary component.
QUAL -> qual:	Qualitative core component of the project (inductive theoretical drive) with a sequential qualitative supplementary component.
QUAN + qual:	Quantitative core component of the project (deductive theoretical drive) with a simultaneous qualitative supplementary component.
QUAN -> qual:	Quantitative core component of the project (deductive theoretical drive) with a sequential qualitative supplementary component.
QUAN + quan:	Quantitative core component of the project (deductive theoretical drive) with a simultaneous quantitative supplementary component.
QUAN -> quan:	Quantitative core component of the project (deductive theoretical drive) with a sequential quantitative supplementary component.

tool used to obtain an enhanced description, explanation, or understanding of the phenomenon as a *strategy*, rather than a *method* complete in itself.[2]

Research projects are conducted either inductively (usually using a qualitative method) or deductively (usually using a quantitative method). In

Box 2: A List of Terms for types of Mixed-Method Design

Component	A phase of the research, driven by the overall direction of the inquiry, during which one or more methodological strategies are used as research tools to address the research question.
Core component of the project	The primary (main) study in which the primary or base method is used to address the research question. This phase of the research is scientifically rigorous.
Method	A cohesive combination of methodological strategies[3] or set of research tools that is inductively or deductively used in conducting qualitative or quantitative inquiry.
Mixed-method design	A plan for a scientifically rigorous research process comprised of a qualitative or quantitative *core component* that directs the theoretical drive, with qualitative or quantitative *supplementary component(s)*. These components of the research fit together to enhance description, understanding and can either be conducted simultaneously or sequentially.
Multi-method design	A plan for a scientifically rigorous *research program* comprised of a series of related qualitative and/or quantitative research projects over time, driven by the *theoretical thrust* of the program. The theoretical drive of an individual project may on occasion counter but not change the overall inductive or deductive direction of the entire program.
Strategy	A methodological research tool, drawn from a qualitative or quantitative method, for addressing the research question by either collecting or analyzing data.
Supplementary component of the project	In this phase of the research, one or more supplementary methodological strategies are used to obtain an enhanced description, understanding or explanation of the phenomenon under investigation. This component of the project can either be conducted at the same time as the core component (simultaneous) or it could follow the core component (sequential). The supplementary component lacks scientific rigor and cannot stand alone.
Theoretical drive	The direction of the inquiry[3] that guides the use of the appropriate qualitative and/or quantitative methodological core. The nature of the research question determines the theoretical drive of a project.
Theoretical thrust	The overall inductive or deductive direction of a research program. The theoretical drive of an individual project may on occasion counter but not change the theoretical thrust of the research program. *© 2006 Janice M. Morse*

mixed-method design, the overall inductive or deductive direction of the inquiry is referred to as the *theoretical drive*, and this encompasses *both* the core and the supplementary components of the project.[3] Also, the theoretical drive of the core component overrides the drive of supplemental component(s). For example, if the design of the project is QUAL±>quan, the theoretical drive is inductive and qualitative, regardless of the minor quantitative supplementary component. Therefore, a mixed-method design *never* has two components of *equal* weighting (i.e., parallel design[2]), nor an "embedded" component, as described by Creswell et al.[4] If a research program (i.e., a series of related projects) involves several mixed-method projects (as in multiple method design), the overall *theoretical thrust* of the program is maintained, even if one of the projects has a theoretical drive countering the theoretical thrust of the program.

Principles for Maintaining Validity in Mixed-Method Design

Mixed-method designs can be challenging to conceive and implement. Three principles ease the process of doing mixed-method design, and assist with maintaining the validity of the project.[3]

Recognize the Role of the Supplementary Strategy

As stated, the rationale for undertaking mixed-method designs is to enhance description or to gain understanding that cannot be obtained using the primary method alone. In the case of QUAL-quan, the role of the supplementary strategy is to provide a "how much" or "how many" to the description of aspects of the phenomenon being studied or to strengthen the implications of the project by quantifying qualitative data (Figure 1). The role of a supplementary strategy in QUAN-qual design is to obtain additional information about aspects of the phenomenon that is necessary to address the research question (Figure 2).

There are essentially three main ways to use supplementary strategies in mixed-method designs:

1) Transform and incorporate supplementary data into the core data set prior to analysis of the data from the core component,
2) Integrate the findings from analyses of a supplementary data set with those of the core method to inform the core component, and
3) Use a supplementary data analysis strategy within a core data set to test emerging hypotheses.

When using supplementary strategies, the researcher must be attentive to the *type and derivation of the sample, sample size*, and *type of data* to prevent threats to validity. It is important that the researcher is clear about the principles and assumptions that underlie both the primary method and the method from which the supplementary strategies are drawn. It is also critical to understand the roles that supplementary strategies can and cannot play. Finally, valid procedures for data collection, transformation, analysis of data, and interpretation of findings are essential.

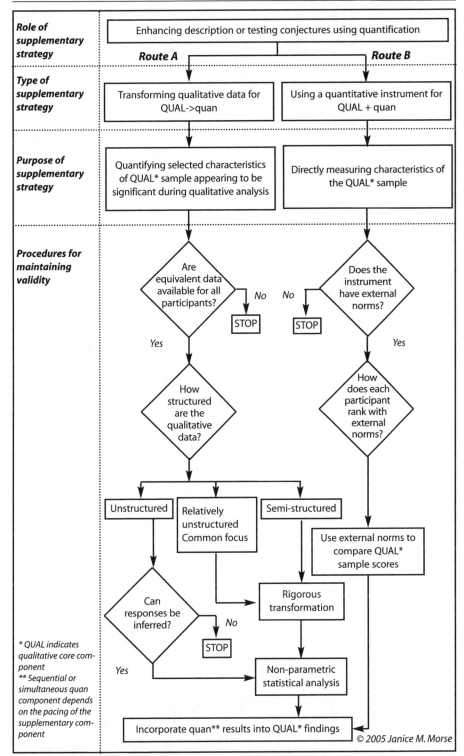

Figure 1: Using supplemental strategies in QUAL ±> quan mixed-method design

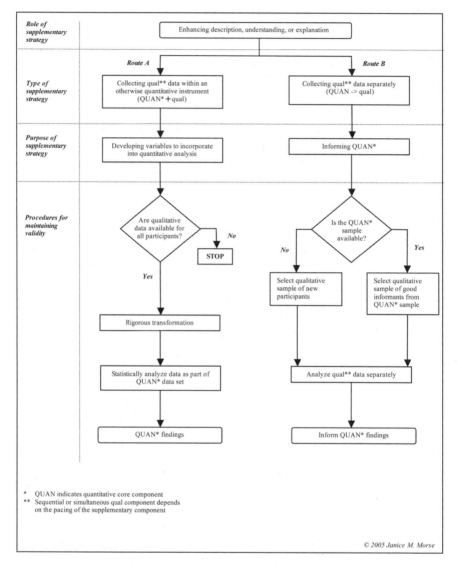

Figure 2: Using supplemental strategies in QUAN ±> qual mixed-method design

Adhere to the Methodological Assumptions of the Primary Method

A researcher should always be aware of the fundamental assumptions of the primary or core method being used, so that in the process of adopting strategies from supplementary methods, the assumptions associated with the core method will not be violated. These assumptions necessarily give rise to design limitations that dictate the nature and types of supplementary research strategies that can be adopted. Prior to embarking on mixed-method design research, the researcher must ask questions such as:

- What is the nature of the phenomenon under investigation?
- Is the nature of the phenomenon being studied in the core and supplementary components of the project the same or different?[5-7]
- If the phenomenon under investigation in the core and supplementary phases of the research is the same, is the phenomenon quantifiable or does it require qualitative exploration?

Questions pertaining to the sample include:

- What is the nature of the primary sample?
- Can the supplementary component of the project use the same sample (or subsample of the study population), or does it require a new sample?
- How will appropriateness and adequacy of a new or supplementary sample be assured?
- Are the analytic assumptions underlying the data involved in the core component of the project and supplementary strategies compatible with one another?[3]

Questions related to data are:

- What is the nature of the data?
- What is the level of the qualitative and quantitative data collected in the core and supplementary components of the project?
- What types of data lend themselves to transformation for QUAL->quan or QUAN + qual?
- How can transformation be done without violating the assumptions of the underlying method?

Work With as Few Data Sets as Possible

Given the nature and scope of the aforementioned issues that must be considered, it is clear that incorporating a supplementary methodological strategy increases the potential threats to validity of a project. Often the knowledge to be gained from additional components is not sufficient to warrant the potential risks to validity. The investigator should assess the research focus and the primary method for completeness by asking where problems in the scope lie, identifying the boundaries of the phenomenon, and evaluating whether or not the results of the project will be generalizable. Since the supplementary component in a mixed-method design is, by definition, incomplete, several supplementary components may result in a hodgepodge of data, analysis and results rather than a comprehensive overall project. In order to maintain coherent findings, all supplementary data sets should remain separate and intact with the exception of a QUAN->qual design. It is vital to note that researchers should have a reason for including each supplementary component while they strive for parsimony and do not forfeit understanding.

Using the above principles, we will now describe and illustrate different types of qualitative and quantitative mixed-method research designs, including procedures for maintaining validity. It is clearly unrealistic to expect that all data, either qualitative or quantitative, could be used in any particular mixed-method design. In the flowcharts for each design, when we reach an operation that we think is impractical or impossible, we have marked this as STOP.

QUAL-quan Mixed-Method Designs

In QUAL-quan designs, the theoretical drive of the core component is inductive. A supplementary strategy is drawn from quantitative methods either during the core component of the project so that qualitative and quantitative methods are carried out simultaneously (QUAL+quan), or following the core component so that qualitative and quantitative methods are carried out sequentially (QUAL->quan). The primary role of a supplementary component in both types of QUAL-quan designs is to enhance description or test conjectures or hypotheses by using quantification (see Figure 1). This can be done by quantifying qualitative characteristics of a sample that appear to be important during analysis (a supplementary data transformation analysis strategy) or by collecting quantitative data about a characteristic of the sample participants (a supplementary data collection strategy). Both approaches are illustrated below, with specific attention where relevant to issues associated with simultaneous or sequential designs.

Threats to validity

The fundamental assumption of qualitative methods is that validity may be threatened by inappropriate quantification. The most important golden rule is *"It must make sense to count whatever is counted."*[8,9] Serendipitous features of the qualitative dataset should not be tabulated. These features include the frequency of words, sentence length and, when the qualitative sample has been purposefully selected, the percentage of participants who identify a particular theme[10] or comprise a category that is meaningless (i.e., it does not contribute to the findings). Similarly, the descriptive "profiling"[8] or "coding"[11] of a qualitative sample is not quantitative data transformation (that is, "quantitizing"[12]). Describing a sample in frequencies and percentages does not alter the nature of the data collected nor the analysis and again, because of the lack of randomization of the sample, does not add to the interpretation of data.

Enhancing QUAL Description by Transforming Qualitative Data for QUAL->quan

This is the most interesting and complex mixed-method design (See Route A, Figure 1). The defining characteristics of the qualitative core method, that is, the attributes that contribute to its validity, are usually at odds with the purpose and assumptions underlying the method from which the supplementary quantitative strategy is drawn. For this reason, transforming qualitative data should always be approached cautiously.

In general, it is best to adopt a design involving transformation of qualitative data at the final stage of a project once solid qualitative results point to directions for formulation and testing of hypotheses, as in a QUAL->quan sequential design. However, most qualitative methods require that data collection and analysis occur simultaneously, driving theoretical sampling. Conjectures worthy of hypothesis formation and testing may therefore emerge at any point in the data collection and analysis process, provided categories are saturated. In this case, in determining appropriate procedures, it is crucial to consider the nature of the sample and amenability of the qualitative data to transformation for statistical analysis.

Often the nature of the qualitative data has inherent characteristics that interfere with or even prohibit the transformation of qualitative data, making it unsuitable for numerical transformation. The researcher should always assess the nature of the qualitative data prior to proceeding with any quantification. As shown in Figure 1 (Route A), a prerequisite for transforming qualitative data is that the same types of data must be obtained from all participants. If, as in some qualitative designs, all informants have not been asked the same questions and data are not equivalent from all participants, it is then not appropriate to transform the qualitative data and the researcher must STOP (Figure 1, Route A). The qualitative core component must stand alone.

On the other hand, where equivalent data are available from all sample participants, decisions about data transformation should be based on 1) theoretical relevance, 2) size and nature of the sample, and 3) type and level of data. Figure 1 (Route A) shows three types of qualitative data that may lend themselves to quantification through data transformation, if handled appropriately. The three types of data collection strategies most common in qualitative research are: unstructured interviews exploring a phenomenon about which little is known in advance (as is used in ethnography); relatively unstructured interviews (including focus group research) exploring a similar event or life experience or stage across participants (e.g., childbirth, breast cancer treatment, or going back to school as a mature adult); and semi-structured interviews or questionnaires seeking more specific information about a phenomenon about which some features are already known.

Since the qualitative sample has been selected purposefully, rather than randomly, it is usually too small to meet the requirements for parametric analysis. The researcher is therefore restricted to non-parametric statistics. Even if the comparison is between two characteristics of participants within the sample, the lack of randomization of the qualitative sample means that generalizability of any quantified results must be regarded with caution.

Unstructured, non-standardized, interviews: Unstructured interviews are common in ethnography, where the investigator learns about the phenomenon in the field as data collection and analysis proceed. In this model, interviewers obtain information from a small number of participants, verify these data, and move on to learn about another aspect of the research phenomenon being explored. Thus, the researcher is considered a "learner in the field" but, more importantly, in this mode of data collection, participants are asked different questions from one another as the study progresses in search of deeper understanding. In general, data from this type of interviewing do not lend themselves to data transformation for the purpose of numerically exporting data for statistical analysis, because data are not equivalent among participants. Should a researcher attempt to numerically code such interviews, it will be evident that the percentage of missing data will render any transformation efforts useless.

If, however, in analysis it becomes clear that the same data *are* available for all participants (even though not intentionally collected to ensure this), and necessary responses may be inferred from data, then it may be possible to proceed with quantification and limited non-parametric statistical analysis (See Figure 1, Route A). These results are then incorporated into findings obtained from the qualitative core component.

Relatively unstructured interviews with a common focus: In the second type of unstructured interview, because the interviews focus on a common event which has inherent stages or processes about which the researcher has some advanced knowledge, it may be possible to code features in the data and to analyze these for all participants quantitatively. For instance, qualitative analysis may result in categories that appear to differentiate participants according to particular attributes (e.g., cultural background and receptivity to hair loss in cancer treatment).

To maximize validity, the researcher must carefully define codes, develop a code book, and establish inter-rater reliability prior to data transformation. The results lend themselves to formulation and testing of emergent hypotheses using non-parametric statistics appropriate to the sample size and level of data. The resulting statistical analysis can be used to enhance the description of qualitative findings and discussion of implications by indicating whether there are significant associations between relevant variables.

Semi-structured interviews/questionnaires: In the third, more structured, type of interview/questionnaire, all participants are asked the same open-ended questions in approximately the same order. Since less in-depth and informative data are obtained from each participant than would be obtained in a study using unstructured interviews, the size of the sample for the primary QUAL method must necessarily be larger (e.g., N=60–100) to compensate for the limited saturation of data categories. Semi-structured interviews/questionnaires pose fewer limitations to data transformation. They allow researchers to code responses numerically, analyze the resulting numerical data, and integrate the findings with qualitative results to enhance conclusions and implications.

As in the previous example, this approach requires defining codes, developing a code book, and establishing inter-rater reliability prior to data transformation (see, for example, Bernard[13]). Each item is then treated as a variable and, depending on the sample size and the level of data, analyzed using parametric or non-parametric statistics. Again, these results are analyzed separately and the results used to enhance the qualitative results.

Enhancing QUAL Description by Collecting Quantitative Data for QUAL+quan

Perhaps the most important and most common QUAL-quan design is qualitatively driven, with a simultaneous quantitative component. The quantitative component employs a standardized instrument as a supplementary strategy to measure quantifiable aspects of the qualitative sample selected in the core component of the research (e.g., answering the question "how much?" about an otherwise qualitative phenomenon such as anxiety). (See Figure 1,

Route B.) It is important to note that this is *not* a data *transformation* process: Data are not transformed from qual to quan or quan to qual in this type of design. This is a relatively straightforward design as long as procedures to maintaining validity are used. First, because the core component requires a small, purposeful sample, rather than the random sample required in quantitative methods, any instrument used with a qualitative sample must have standardized norms against which the researcher can compare the obtained scores. Because of the intentional bias of the qualitative sample, scores are virtually meaningless in the absence of such external norms. If an appropriate standardized instrument cannot be located, the researcher has no choice but to draw a larger and adequate sample that is comparative, or STOP (See Figure 1, Route B).

Second, if a researcher needs to measure some quantifiable aspects of a phenomenon once the qualitative core project is already completed (as in the sequential design), a sampling problem may occur because the original participants in the qualitative sample may no longer be located. Is it legitimate to administer the quantitative instrument to another equivalent purposefully selected, qualitative sample? Yes, provided the same criteria for its selection are used. The same contingencies for interpreting the scores as in the simultaneous QUAL-quan design holds. Since the sample remains small and purposefully chosen (for instance, there are only six heart-lung transplant patients in the region this year), external norms must be used to interpret the scores obtained.

While these considerations are important, if the instrument is appropriate for the purpose and has standardized norms, there is no inherent threat to validity in this design. The quantitative supplementary data may be used in two ways: (1) Each individual's score may be used in the descriptive profiling of each participant, or (2) the data sets may be analyzed separately and the results of the quan supplementary strategy used to enhance description of the findings of the primary QUAL method by incorporating such useful information. For instance, a researcher may note, "the participants in the study were so anxious that their scores on the anxiety scale were 2 standard deviations above the mean of the standardized population."

QUAN-qual Mixed-Method Designs

Because quantitative methods are usually used when a reasonable amount is already known about a phenomenon, QUAN-qual designs are less common. They are almost invariably planned at the proposal stage because some aspect of the phenomenon to be studied does not lend itself to quantification, yet the investigators wish to include information about that particular aspect.

The primary role of supplementary methods in QUAN-qual mixed-method designs is to enhance description, understanding, or explanation about the phenomenon that the primary method cannot access. This may be accomplished by either a) collecting qualitative data using open-ended questions within an otherwise structured instrument, or b) collecting and analyzing qualitative data separately to explain puzzling quantitative findings. Both of these roles are illustrated in Figure 2, along with special considerations, where relevant, specific to simultaneous and sequential designs.

Enhancing QUAN Description, Understanding, or Explanation by Collecting Qualitative Data Within a Quantitative Instrument (Quan + qual)

The most common way in which supplementary qualitative data are obtained in a mixed-method design is by intentionally including semi-structured, open-ended questions within or at the end of a structured questionnaire. Even when the qualitative data are solicited systematically in this way, the large randomly selected quantitative sample is cumbersome for qualitative purposes. Therefore qualitative data obtained as part of an otherwise quantitative instrument or questionnaire must be used cautiously to avoid threats to validity. The sample (both selection and size) for the qualitative data is the same as for the primary quantitative method (i.e., large and randomly selected); therefore, quantification of the qualitative data are possible. The textual responses may be analyzed by coding to transform and import these codes into the quantitative data set as variables, consistent with the QUAN theoretical drive of the project. The procedures for maintaining validity are similar to those for semi-structured interviews/questionnaires: codes are defined, a code book developed, and inter-rater reliability is then established and periodically re-checked throughout the coding procedures.

Although some researchers do code and analyze unsolicited comments written by respondents in the margins of a quantitative questionnaire, this should not be considered an appropriate supplementary strategy. These data are not available for all participants, therefore requiring that the researcher STOP. Perhaps even more importantly such data may be indicative of problems with the validity of an instrument and may require the researcher to start the project again, using a qualitative method if a more suitable instrument cannot be located or developed.

Enhancing QUAN Description, Understanding, or Explanation by Collecting Qualitative Data Separately (Quan -> qual)

In a sequential design, once the quantitative analysis is completed, supplementary qualitative data collection may be necessary to investigate an unexpected or unexplainable finding prior to drawing conclusions. Sampling in such cases is trickier. Some investigators randomly select a qualitative sample from the quantitative participants, while others purposefully select participants according to criteria developed from the quantitative data, such as participants scoring in a certain range on an instrument, or demographic characteristics. While the intent of investigators using these methods of selection is to ensure a "balanced sample," in actual fact such strategies do not ensure that the participants will meet the criteria of "good informants," a standard requirement of qualitative methods. These practices violate the principles underlying sampling in qualitative methods. A qualitative sample of good informants should be selected from the QUAN sample (See Figure 2).[14]

Again, in this research design, the qualitative supplementary component does not have the level of development (that is, saturation, analytic development, or scope) of a complete qualitative project. Qualitative data collected as a supplementary strategy in this sequential design are not transformed into quantified data or variables, but the findings are incorporated into the discussion of quantitative results to add explanation.

Conclusion

In this chapter, we have discussed the major mixed-method designs. These designs are not meant to be conclusive, but rather to illustrate the risks to validity and recommend procedures for preventing threats to validity. There are other mixed-method designs that we have not addressed, for instance, QUAL-qual and QUAN-quan designs because they do not have the same methodological problems.

The principles identified here are central for conducting mixed-method design research, explicating the role of the supplementary strategy, respecting the methodological assumptions of the primary method, working with as few data sets as possible, and clarifying the need for necessary procedures when conducting rigorous mixed-method research. We identified procedures for combining methods from apparently incompatible paradigms, and allowing them to co-exist without threatening validity. The primary contribution of this chapter is the explication of the necessary steps in Figures 1 and 2, to move through the mixed-method procedures including data transformation for various types of qualitative data.

Summary Points
- Mixed-method designs offer unique and important contributions, and should be implemented with careful attention to preventing threats to validity.
- Researchers should have a reason for including each supplementary component while they strive for parsimony and do not forfeit understanding.
- Three principles assist with maintaining the validity of the project: recognize the role of the supplementary strategy, adhere to the methodological assumptions of the primary method, and work with as few data sets as possible.
- The fundamental assumption of qualitative methods is that validity may be threatened by inappropriate quantification. The most important golden rule is *"It must make sense to count whatever is counted."*

References

1) Morse, J.M. Approaches to Qualitative-Quantitative Methodological Triangulation. *Nursing Research*. 1991; 40:120-123.

2) There is no consensus on terminology. See, for example: Teddlie, C. and Tashakkori, A. Major Issues and Controversies in the Use of Mixed Methods in the Social and Behavioral Sciences. In Tashakkori, A. and Teddlie, C. (Eds.). *Handbook of Mixed Methods in Social and Behavioral Research*. Thousand Oaks: Sage Publications, 2003, pp. 3-50.

3) Morse, J.M. Principles of Mixed Methods and Multimethod Research Design. In Tashakkori, A. and Teddlie, C. (Eds.). *Handbook of Mixed Methods in Social and Behavioral Research*. Thousand Oaks: Sage Publications, 2003, pp. 189-208.

4) Creswell, J.W., Clark, V.L.P., Gutmann, M.L., and Hanson, W.E. Advanced Mixed Methods Research Designs. In Tashakkori, A. and Teddlie, C. (Eds.). *Handbook of Mixed Methods in Social and Behavioral Research*. Thousand Oaks: Sage Publications, 2003, pp. 209-240.

5) Sim, J. and Sharp, K. A Critical Appraisal of the Role of Triangulation in Nursing Research. *International Journal of Nursing Studies*. 1998; 35:23-31.

6) Sale, J.E.M., Lohfeld, L.H., and Brazil, K. Revisiting the Quantitative-Qualitative Debate: Implications for Mixed-Methods Research. *Quality & Quantity*. 2002; 36:43-53.

7) Erzberger, C. and Prein, G. Triangulation: Validity and Empirically-Based Hypothesis Construction. *Quality & Quantity*. 1997; 31:141-154.

8) Sandelowski, M. Real Qualitative Researchers Do Not Count: The Use of Numbers in Qualitative Research. *Research in Nursing and Health*. 2001; 24:230-240.

9) Sandelowski, M. Tables or Tableaux? The Challenges of Writing and Reading Mixed Methods Studies. In Tashakkori, A. and Teddlie, C. (Eds.). *Handbook of Mixed Methods in Social and Behavioral Research*. Thousand Oaks: Sage Publications, 2003, pp. 321-350.

10) Onwuegbuzie, A.J. and Teddlie, C. A Framework for Analyzing Data in Mixed Methods Research. In Tashakkori, A. and Teddlie, C. (Eds.). *Handbook of Mixed Methods in Social and Behavioral Research*. Thousand Oaks: Sage Publications, 2003, pp. 351-384.

11) Morse, J.M. and Richards, L. *Read Me First for a User's Guide to Qualitative Methods*. Thousand Oaks, CA: Sage Publications, 2002.

12) Tashakkori, A. and Teddlie, C. *Mixed Methodology: Combining Qualitative and Quantitative Approaches*. Vol 46. Thousand Oaks: Sage Publications, 1998.

13) Bernard, H.R. *Social Research Methods. Qualitative and Quantitative Approaches*. Thousand Oaks, CA: Sage Publications, 2000.

14) Spradley, J. *The Ethnographic Interview*. New York: Holt, Rinehart and Winston, 1979.

Acknowledgements: This work has been funded through a doctoral fellowship to Ruth Wolfe as a fellow in a CIHR Strategic Training Initiative in Health Research (EQUIPP) at the International Institute for Qualitative Methodology, University of Alberta.

Chapter 7

If Not, Why Not?
Synchronizing Qualitative and Quantitative Research in Studying the Elderly

Jay Sokolovsky, PhD

Introduction

One of the key areas of research dealing with health and aging is social networks.[1,2] The study of social networks provides ways to understand how health information, interpersonal support, and the exchange of goods and services often proceed. Furthermore, the variety of social network organization reveals differences and disparities among communities that need to be better appreciated. This topic not only has produced a rich, diverse literature but has also revealed conflicting and contradictory findings.

While a concern for qualitative aspects of social networks of elderly populations is sometimes addressed in study design, it is seldom fused with quantitative measures throughout the entire project. All too often, qualitative measures are considered a separate, adjunct part of methodology, and are not used to influence the construction of other kinds of variables. Not only is this integration important for producing a clear understanding of the complex nature, meaning, and impact of social networks on health, but qualitative approaches to research design are critical for creating appropriate quantitative measures, as well. This is to say *both* qualitative and quantitative variables are necessary for a complex understanding of the interface between social networks and health.

Moreover, the social and cultural context in which measured variables exist and are produced is very rarely examined, even in qualitative studies. This is particularly critical in examining health disparity between ethnic communities which are frequently essentialized as racial groups. The erasing of diversity within groups is empirically captured by terms such as Hispanic or Asian. Terms like these reduce the complexity inherent in communities.

As a way to help resolve some of these issues, this chapter first reviews some of the theoretical issues involved with the study of social networks and aging, then presents an "Ethnometric Social Network" strategy. This procedure has been used in several studies to effectively integrate qualitative and quantitative approaches and maximize the strengths of each methodology.

Quantitative and Qualitative Methods: Separate but Equal?

Over the past two decades a multidisciplinary movement sometimes referred to as "Qualitative Gerontology" has attempted to establish qualitative modes of analysis as an equal partner to more quantitative methods.[3] One of its strongest advocates is sociologist Jaber Gubrium who has argued that qualitative approaches should not be viewed as a second-class precursor to more "powerful" statistical analysis.[4] According to Gubrium, good qualitative research is important to the generation of theoretically informed findings. Such work attempts to represent the "native complexity" of behavior and how that complexity is organized.[5-8] By using a relatively small number of cases, it is possible to retain a picture of the qualitative nature of sociocultural variables *and* process. At the same time this approach strives to avoid overly simple theoretical models.

However, relying entirely on a qualitative approach has the potential problem of providing depth only about a local and highly circumscribed universe. This focus on the small scale restricts the application of ethnographic results beyond the study sites, such as a particular type of nursing facility, segment of an ethnic community, or category of individual, such as older homeless women in New York City shelters. Even worse, it can blind researchers to important processes and issues related to a comprehensive understanding of health inequalities.

For example, the qualitative and ethnographic study of African American elderly has shown the tremendous potential for extended kin and community-based support centered in such institutions as the church.[9] This has led to the assumption within the African American community as well as among researchers that this population makes comparatively little use of formal long-term care facilities such as nursing homes. However, in fusing an intensive focus group approach with quantitative studies, Groger and Mayberry[10] have seriously challenged this assumption. The authors showed that not only were young African American adults in Ohio misunderstanding their family's capacity for informal long-term care, but this ethnic group had higher per capita nursing home usage than populations labeled "white." In other words, the interplay of comparative, survey data with family level information revealed an aspect of social support of elders which had been missed by focusing on qualitative variables alone.

Social Networks, Aging, and Well-Being

The use of social networks to study the lives of the elderly and examine their place in varying social systems has flourished over the last two decades.[11,12] This interest derived from a natural connection to the theoretical ideas of "disengagement," "activity," and "exchange" models which sought to account for the patterns by which older adults construct a social world and transform it in relation to the demands of aging. Each model has been used to try to predict how patterns of personal social engagement relate to operationalized measures of well-being, life satisfaction, or morale.[13] However, in attempting to measure social relationships associated with the "network" idea, particularly in the applied realm, analysts have focused more on the mechanical rudiments of personal networks. This has been used especially to detail the individual components of "support systems". These data are typically abstracted from reported exchanges of the elderly with their social others, often by asking, "If you had this type of problem, who would you turn to?" Thus, numerous studies have tried to ascertain correlates of well-being measures with discrete parts of network systems in order to determine which kind of social link—kin ties, friends, or agency supports—is more correlated with well-being.

The major problem of this procedure has been the general failure to treat social support network variables as multidimensional constructs that can reveal important aspects of process. While variables such as marital status, living arrangements, and number of children often serve as surrogate measures for social support networks, various studies show the need to go beyond such simplistic measures of network and support. For example, analysis of the Social Networks in Adult Life survey shows that the qualities of support are more consistent predictors of life satisfaction than measures of quantity.[14] While the mere existence of a family member or a friend in a network was not significantly related to well-being, satisfaction with these relationships was. Furthermore, ties with friends tend to have a positive effect on individual satisfaction with a person's network, and are much less likely to have a negative effect. The reverse was true for kin ties (for an international perspective see Antonucci, Okorodudu, and Akiyama[15]).

Problems in Survey Approaches to Social Networks

These studies address a key problem in survey approaches to social networks. Because people live within networks that contain many types of relationships *at the same time*, isolating each sector for analysis may provide a false sense of understanding of how social relations impact people's lives. Many researchers may have indulged in a basic illusion while conducting such research. By focusing on the "personal" exchanges of a discrete group of elderly, researchers often become convinced that the detailed look at dyadic interchange provides access to the most immediate realm for understanding the quality of life the aged engage in. What may be missed, however, is how the bits of interaction connect to the whole of a social matrix and how these bonds exist in the community and the cultural system which gives social action real meaning over the life cycle. This basic problem may be why there has been such confounding information about social interaction and the perceived quality of life of the aged.

The difficulty understanding the significance of statistical survey variables appears prominently in the analysis of social interaction and support in ethnic family and neighborhood contexts. As such studies show the predominant use of so-called sociometric techniques for gathering data, it is sometimes quite difficult to know the meaning of statistically significant differences or the lack of such variation. For example, in the "Social and Cultural Contexts of Aging" study conducted in Los Angeles,[16] social interaction with children, grandchildren, other relatives, and friends were compared among whites, blacks, and Mexican-Americans. White elderly were considerably less likely than Mexican-Americans to see children and grandchildren on a weekly basis although no difference was found for contact with other relatives. On the other hand, Mexican-Americans saw friends and neighbors less frequently. Older blacks and whites were shown to have almost identical frequency of contact with grandchildren or other relatives although smaller percentages of blacks reported seeing children and neighborhood friends frequently.

Using these quantitative bits of data to understand the health issues of the aged in familial and community networks is problematic. A study in San Diego added to the Los Angeles findings noted above to reveal that even Hispanics who lived alone had four times more extended kin in the local area than whites. At the same time, they also found that these individuals "suffered in silence," and were *less* likely to turn to family members in times of need[17] (p. 392). The consequences of this behavior appear to be high levels of alienation, low life satisfaction, and other psychological problems. Part of the difficulty stems from unmet expectations of family interaction. More recent longitudinal work among barrio dwelling Mexican Americans in San Antonio, Texas, showed that the number of children was not associated with reported caregiver availability. In fact, elders with the greatest need for a caregiver were the most likely to report that one was not available.[18] Even in the previously mentioned studies in Los Angeles, which showed high levels of family interaction and general support for elderly Hispanic-Americans, these aged were more likely to display symptoms of mental stress than either whites or blacks. In both locales the main sources of concern were children and family. Of particular concern from a health disparity perspective is that some studies have shown that Hispanic-Americans families, when compared to other ethnic groups surveyed, use community-based services at a very low rate.[19,20] In other words, some groups of Hispanic elders face the dilemma of lacking appropriate health supports within large family networks, yet fail to make substantial use of available formal health service resources.

Addressing the general issue of family network ties, the Bengtson and Morgan Los Angeles study above found that approximately 40 percent of both whites and blacks in Los Angeles see "grandchildren" and "other relatives" weekly.[16] However, this finding does not mean that the two sets of aged connect to kinship networks and access resources by such ties in the same way. Other studies, such as that by Gibson[21] or Nellie Tate,[22] have provided clues to some health care related differences. For example, older black women are four times more likely than older white females to live with young dependent relatives under eighteen years of age. Therefore, while a simple network variable shows little variation, the *process* by which multigenerational households form can be quite different: it is the young who join the household of black female elders versus the reverse that tends to occur in Euro-American families. In Philadelphia's urban context Tate[22] found that the former path of multigenerational household formation produced more psychological acceptance of higher levels of functional impairment related to chronic illness among elders. Such studies highlight the critical need to look at both the process of network formation and how it functions as a whole entity.

Understanding Social Networks as Complex Whole Constructs

This issue of treating social networks as complex, whole constructs has not been totally ignored. The work of Wenger in rural Wales[23,24] and comparative work by Francis in the United States and England[25] are two important projects that indicate the potential richness of this approach. Both studies indicate that network variables which assess total network morphology and the quality of exchanges are the best indicators of well-being among the elderly and among their caregivers. Wenger's longitudinal research demonstrated how the structure and degree of integration of social networks was vitally related, not only to the provision of informal helping directed toward an elder but to other indicators of well-being, as well. Wenger found that the network type classified as "locally integrated"—which fused active family, friend, and neighbor ties with church and other voluntary organizations —was the most associated with network support, independent functioning, and high morale.[24] The other network types noted were: local self-contained; wider community focused; and private restricted. In a specific study of family caregivers for relatives with dementia, she found that only locally integrated network structures or those transformed into what she cataloged as "local, family centered" support systems could effectively cope with long-term care.[23]

In *Will You Still Need Me Will You Still Feed Me When I'm 84*[25], Doris Francis shows how the dialectic between situational context (e.g., residential stability) and the way kin and neighbor networks are intertwined over time relates to the formation of supportive communities in late adulthood. In a comparison between Jews from Cleveland and Leeds, England, she examined how the migration histories, the impact of housing policy, and community organization altered the structure and communication within whole networks. In the U.S. sample she found that networks as a whole have less deep connection into the community. Furthermore, while elders seem psychologically attached to their kin ties, they have a very unrealistic understanding of these relations and the nature of the exchange that actually goes on. Francis related this finding to the lack of balance and interconnection of community networks with close kin ties in Cleveland. This was very different than the case in England where the social connections with which elders entered old age were much more stable and intertwined in the lives of a wider variety of network players. This study shows how community context can powerfully alter not only the structure and depth of network configurations but also their psychological valence.

Developing an Ethnometric Approach to the Dilemma of Rigor vs. Relevance

It is important to note that the studies by Wenger and Francis take very different approaches to gathering network data on the elderly.[23-25] The former used a relatively simple questionnaire (sample sizes numbered a few hundred) embedded in a generalized community study, while the latter used a highly intensive life history approach (sample sizes were several dozen) coupled with long-term ethnographic research. These studies tread the pathway between rigor and relevance and reveal some weaknesses. The first study downplays creating complex network variables, and the second study lacks the ability to generate substantial sample sizes. To resolve this dilemma, I developed what I call an "ethnometric" social network approach, integrating ethnographically focused "Network Profiles" into survey-based interview protocols with sample sizes of 2–300 persons (See Sokolovsky 1986 for a full discussion of Network Profiles).[11]

This approach to examining social networks involves not only ethnographically defining the transactional nature and community context of social linkages, but also delineating the cultural meaning they hold for social actors. The approach was initially developed through work with Belleview Hospital and later with DownState Medical Center, in one of the early studies of released mental hospital patients released to Single Room Occupancy (SRO) hotels in New York City during the early and mid-1970s. The author and Carl Cohen, a community psychiatrist with training in sociology, developed a strategy that combined anthropological and clinical data to look at a sample of 44 individuals in a single hotel. The approach was further refined and integrated with quantitative survey instruments in longitudinal, health-focused studies of elderly populations in these same kinds of environments and of older homeless men and women throughout New York City.[26]

The initial research focus which stimulated this methodological approach was the extent to which the social worlds constructed by "independently" living persons labeled as schizophrenic, influenced their ability to survive in a non-institutional environment. Among the findings this research demonstrated were that: (1) very few schizophrenics in this environment were truly socially isolated; (2) the size as well as the quality and morphology of networks had an impact on survival in the community; (3) the interface of the informal and formal support systems was a crucial factor in influencing how people coped in mid-Manhattan; and (4) understanding the process by which networks were formed, sustained, and eventually dissipated was as crucial to understanding links to mental health as were the structural aspects of the networks themselves.[27] A key issue which became clear in subsequent studies was the capacity, or lack thereof, of the local urban environment to be a medium for supportive social connections that can promote health care. Understanding this last factor requires the long-term involvement of qualitative methodologies that focus on process.

The Ethnometric Approach

Establishing Cultural Relevance

The ethnometric approach and the Network Analysis Profile (NAP) developed in this research was an attempt to deal with the constant methodological battle of rigor versus relevance in the quest for articulating the study of health with explanatory models of behavior and adaptation. This problem was addressed by establishing the ethnographically relevant frames of behavior within which transactions occur and then creating network profiles to elicit comparable data between respondents in a sample. For example, the use of seemingly straightforward eliciting frames such as, "How many friends do you have?" would often result in people either claiming to be friends with everyone or the statement that, "I'm a loner, I don't need no one and no one needs me." Survey interviews in SRO environments in Seattle echoed this sentiment and caused Lally, Black, Thornock, and Hawkins[28] to depict elderly women in these places as having only limited functional ties with hotel staff and nearby business proprietors. Their respondents "consistently claimed to neither be friends with or even know other women in their hotels" (p. 70). Had my work been based on survey interviews alone instead of qualitative fieldwork, I might have come to a similar conclusion. The research strategy provided a way to see that in the New York SROs, no elders had friendly ties to everyone, and the self-proclaimed "loners" were as likely as not to have social support networks larger than the mean for the sample.

Who are "Friends"?

The issue of "friends" became even more problematic in studying the homeless elderly as we found that the middle-class understanding of friendship had limited cultural meaning for this population. Instead of friend, they used the term "associate" to manage and discuss the world of non-kin and non-agency ties[26]. A typical construction of this idea was expressed by an elderly homeless ex-painter, "Here, you can't have real friends when you're old, …you only have friends from your childhood. If they are lost, friends are gone, and you just have some associates" (p. 122). However, as in the case of our SRO research, being on the street and observing the daily lives of Skid Row's oldest adults showed that marginality did not mean total isolation. Rather, their lives were based on the careful manipulation of a highly fluid set of social ties trusted just enough to help accomplish the tasks necessary for survival.

The NAP

The NAP evolved out of these research settings in an effort to distill the best elements of the sociological and anthropological approaches to examining social networks. In general, the former approach employed less detailed sociometrics that were capable of yielding large samples, whereas the latter approach examined more complex measures of interaction but consequently studied fewer subjects. The NAP was also designed to elicit both objective (behavioral) and subjective (affectual) measures of social interaction. The NAP is a semi-structured instrument that examines several fields of social interaction between a focus person and his or her social world. These include: household/kinship linkages; non-kin linkages (neighbors, friends); and formal linkages (agency staff, clergy, health care professionals, etc.). Within each field of interaction, lists of important persons are compiled, and information is gathered about *network member attributes* (age, gender, ethnicity, location, work status); *network linkage attributes* (contact frequency, types/quality of exchange); and *network structure attributes* (size, density, gender/age/ethnic homogeneity, connections between network components, general network morphology). Persons were included in the social network if they were in contact with the respondent (i.e., through a material exchange, social activity, or 15-minute conversation) over the three months prior to interview (12 months for outside nonkin and kin). Significant persons could be included if they had been in contact with the respondent in the previous 12 months. The keys to this approach include (1) anchoring data requests in concrete and culturally meaningful categories developed from at least 2–3 months of community based fieldwork; (2) including some information redundancy to cross-check responses; (3) holding regular meetings with the full research staff to be able to modify the survey protocol based on a trial phase of ethnographic fieldwork.

The CARE Survey

The structured survey questionnaire chosen for projects was The Comprehensive Assessment and Referral Evaluation (CARE). The CARE was developed by Barry Gurland and his associates[29] in the mid-1970s and was designed to assess the level of physical health, psychiatric symptoms, and social and economic needs of geriatric populations. It was the principal instrument used in their Cross-National Study of elderly persons living in New York City and London.

Both the CARE and NAP were designed to be administered by persons with little or no previous expertise in research, aging, health care, or social services. In fact, previous findings indicated that specialization sometimes created problems for interviewers who might inadvertently interject their professional styles into the interview. Thus, a clinical psychologist might evoke an excessive emotional response, or a physician might elicit an excessive number of physical complaints. Moreover, the professional demeanor can create a distancing and wary response from a population that is suspicious and cynical about experts and service providers.

The initial training sessions for the NAP and CARE were typically completed over two and four days, respectively. Training consisted of a detailed review of the instruments followed by scoring of video and audiotapes and the interviewing of each other. Once the project began, the interviewers audio taped the first three interviews for which permission was granted and then every tenth interview. These and the completed questionnaire were reviewed for accuracy. In addition, the project staff reviewed all completed questionnaires as they were returned.

In addition to conducting the NAP and CARE, traditional fieldwork was carried out that centered on participant observation, life history collection, and intensive interviews that took place over the course of many months. Finally, an assessment of the ethnographic data was conducted at each project's mid-points to check if there were any key parts of our population that we missed.

Conclusions

Despite the difficulties of fully integrating qualitative and quantitative research in gerontological research, it is necessary to seriously ask the question, "If not, why not?" with respect to the integration of qualitative and quantitative research methods and design. Several decades of studies have demonstrated that qualitatively constructed variables often have the most impact on understanding the kinds of health issues critical to the life of the elderly. It is therefore incumbent on qualitative researchers to understand how their contributions to methodology and data can be appreciated both on their own *and* in collaboration with more quantified means of understanding reality. Without the added value of embedding such work within a more quantitatively constructed frame, all too often we are left with a "just so story," which may prompt us to ask, "So what?" The approach suggested in this chapter will help illuminate important areas of health and aging research and in so doing open new and compelling questions to pursue.

Summary Points
- Integration of qualitative and quantitative methods is important for producing a clear understanding of the complex nature, meaning, and impact of social networks on health, as well as for creating appropriate quantitative measures.
- Social support network variables are multidimensional constructs that can reveal important aspects of process; network variables which assess total network morphology and the quality of exchanges are the best indicators of well-being.
- Qualitative researchers must understand how their contributions to methodology and data can be appreciated both on their own *and* in collaboration with more quantified means of understanding reality.

References

1) Bosworth, H. and Schaie, K. The Relationship of Social Environment, Social Network and Health Outcomes in the Seattle Longitudinal Study: Two Analytical Approaches. *Journal of Gerontology: Psychological Services.* 1997; 52B(5):197-205.
2) Michael, Y., Colditz, G., Coakley, E., and Kawachi, I. Health Behaviors, Social Networks, and Healthy Aging: Cross-Sectional Evidence from the Nurses' Health Study. *Quality of Life Research.* 1999; 8,711-722.
3) Gubrium, J. and Sankar, A., eds. *Qualitative Methods in Aging Research.* Sage: Newbury Park, CA; 1994.

4) Gubrium, J. Qualitative Research Comes of Age in Gerontology. *Gerontologist.* 1992; 32:5:581-582.

5) Rubinstein, R. Anthropological Methods in Gerontological Research: Entering the Realm of Meaning. *Journal of Aging Studies.* 1992; 6:57-66.

6) _____. The Engagement of Life History and Life Review Among the Aged: A Research Case Study. *Journal of Aging Studies.* 1995; 9(3):187-203.

7) Luborsky, M. Creative Challenges and the Construction of Meaningful Life Narratives. In C. Adams-Price (ed.), *Creativity and Successful Aging: Theoretical and Empirical Approaches.* New York: Springer. 1998: 311-337.

8) Rowles, Graham and Schoenberg, Nancy (eds.), *Qualitative Gerontology: Perspectives for a New Century.* New York: Springer, 2002.

9) Peterson, J. Age of Wisdom: Elderly Black Women in Family and Church. In Sokolovsky, J. (ed.), *The Cultural Context of Aging Worldwide Perspectives,* 2nd ed., Westport, CT: Greenwood, 1997; 276-93.

10) Groger, L. and Mayberry, P. Caring Too Much: Cultural Lag in African American's Perceptions of Filial Responsibilities. *Journal of Cross-Cultural Gerontology.* 2001; 16:1:21-39,

11) Sokolovsky, J., Network Methodologies in the Study of Aging. In: Fry, C. and Keith, J. (eds.), *New Methods for Old Age Research,* 2nd edition, Boston: Bergin and Garvey, 1986; 231-261.

12) Wenger, C. Review of Findings on Support Networks of Older Europeans. *Journal of Cross-Cultural Gerontology.* 1997; 2:1:1–21.

13) Lee, G. Theoretical Perspective on Social Networks. In: Sauer, W. and Coward, R. (eds.), *Social Support Networks and the Care of the Elderly.* New York: Springer; 1985: 21-27.

14) Antonucci, T. and Akiyama, H. Convoys of Social Relations: Family and Friendships Within a Life Span Context. In: Bleisner, R. and Bedford, B., (eds.), *Handbook of Aging and the Family.* New York, NY: Greenwood; 1995: 355-371.

15) Antonucci, T., Okorodudu, C., and Akiyama, H. International Perspectives on the Well-Being of Older Adults. *Journal of Social Issues.* 2002; 58:4.

16) Bengtson, V. and Morgan, L. Ethnicity and Aging: A Comparison of Three Ethnic Groups. In: Sokolovsky, J., (ed.), *Growing Old in Different Societies: Cross-Cultural Perspectives.* Acton, MA: Copley. 1987: 157-167.

17) Weeks, J. and Cuellar, J. The Role of Family Members in the Helping Networks of Older People. *Gerontologist.* 1981; 1:338-94.

18) Markides, K.S., Black, S.A. Aging and Health Behaviors in Mexican Americans. *Family and Community Health,* 19:11-18, 1996.

19) Mui, A. and Burnette, M. Long-Term Care Service use by Frail Elders: Is Ethnicity a Factor? *Gerontologist.* 1994; 34:2:190-198.

20) Valle, R., Yamada, A., and Barrio, C. Ethnic Differences in Social Network Help-Seeking Strategies Among Latino and Euro-American Dementia Caregivers. *Aging and Mental Health.* 2004; 8:6:535-543.

21) Gibson, R. Promoting Successful and Productive Aging in Minority Populations. In: Bond, L.A., Cutler, S.J., and Grams, A. (eds.), *Promoting Successful and Productive Aging.* Thousand Oaks, CA: Sage; 1995: 279-288.

22) Tate, N. The Black Aging Experience. In: McNeely, R. and Olen, J., (eds.), *Aging in Minority Groups..* Beverly Hills: Sage: 1983.

23) Wenger, C. *Support Networks and Dementia: Ageing in Liverpool: Working Paper 4,* Centre for Social Policy Research and Development, Bangor, Wales: University of Wales, 1992.

24) Wenger, C. The Formation of Social Networks: Self-Help, Mutual Aid and Old People in Contemporary Britain. *Journal of Aging Studies.* 1993; 25-40.

25) Francis, D. 1984. *Will You Still Need Me, Will You Still Feed Me When I'm 84?* Bloomington, IN: Indiana University Press.

26) Cohen, C. and Sokolovsky, J. *Old Men of the Bowery: Survival Strategies of the Homeless,* New York: Guilford Press; 1989. *Psychological Services;* 1997; 52B(5): 197-205.

27) Sokolovsky, J., Cohn, C., Berger, D., and Geiger, J. Personal Networks of Ex-Mental Patients in a Manhattan SRO hotel, *Human Organization.* 1978; 37:1:4-15.

28) Lally, M, Black, E., Thornock M., and Hawkins, J.D. Older Women in Single-Room Occupant (SRO) Hotels: A Seattle Profile. *Gerontologist,* 1979; 19:67-73.

29) Gurland, L., Kuriansky, J., Sharpe, L., et al. The Comprehensive Assessment and Referral Evaluation (CARE): Rationale, Development, and Reliability. *International Journal of Aging and Human Development.* 1977; 8:9-42

Chapter 8

Codes to Theory: A Critical Stage in Qualitative Analysis

Elizabeth H. Bradley, PhD and Leslie A. Curry, PhD, MPH

Introduction

The use of qualitative research methodologies in clinical medicine, nursing, public health, and health services research has grown substantially in the last decade. Applications are highly diverse and include, but are not limited to, studies of culture change,[1,2] diffusion of innovations and quality improvement strategies,[3-5] and novel interventions to improve care.[6,7] With increased use of qualitative approaches, several important methodological papers[8-10] have augmented seminal texts[11-15] to provide guidance to researchers seeking to ensure the quality and rigor of their qualitative studies. Nevertheless, while principles and mechanics of coding qualitative data have been described[12-13,15-18] and stages of data analysis have been enumerated,[11,19] there has been less attention paid to the process of integrating coded qualitative data to develop theory. Theoretical development is a critical and unique contribution of qualitative research. Accordingly, this chapter describes common strategies for moving between the codes and the theory, in order to assist researchers in generating valuable insights from qualitative studies.

This chapter is organized in five parts. First, we provide a brief overview of fundamental principles and steps in qualitative data analysis. Second, we discuss the process of developing coding schemes and coding data. Third, we review how coded data can be used to produce taxonomies, key themes, and/or conceptual models. In this section, we also present examples of these theoretical products. Fourth, we offer a set of techniques to enhance the validity and reliability of the process of moving from the codes to the theory. The last section summarizes the central concepts presented in the chapter.

Principles of and Steps in Qualitative Data Analysis

Principles of Analysis

Qualitative analysis is an ongoing and iterative process, which is not sharply divided from data collection and formulation or revision of research questions. Unlike quantitative studies, in which data collection is generally completed before data analysis begins, qualitative analysis is most effective when it occurs simultaneously throughout data collection. This analytic approach allows for continual reflection, memo writing, and refining of

91

research questions over the course of the study. Because of the integrative and flexible nature of qualitative analysis, it is critical to document analytic decisions with an audit trail.[12] The audit trail may include memos written by researchers as they develop themes and connections in the data, revise coding schemes, define and refine various codes and their properties, and develop hypotheses or conceptual models.

Steps in Analysis

Steps in qualitative analysis with the goal of theoretical development include: preparing the data, reviewing the data for general understanding, coding the data, analyzing the data, and developing theory. Preparing the data refers to synthesizing data into transcripts or test-based notes that can be reviewed by the research team. For instance, in a focus group study, preparing the data would involve transcribing and checking the transcription of the audio taped material or hand-written notes and creating documents specific to each interview or group. Careful formatting, including labeling transcripts with a systematic file name and inserting line-numbering facilitates communication among members of the analysis team about sections of the interviews. Once prepared, transcripts should be read closely to gain a general understanding of the data. At this stage, it is important to pay attention to the overall tone and identify key ideas in the interviews, without coding for conceptual content. This step is important, as seeing the whole can promote better understanding of specific concepts noted during detailed coding. The next steps are coding and analysis, which help categorize voluminous open-ended data into a set of homogeneous and exhaustive concepts. In this often very time-consuming stage, a coding scheme is created, applied, and refined as indicated by the data. Analysis continues in this iterative fashion until "theoretical saturation" is achieved.[13] The last step, developing theory, refers to the synthesis and integration of the coded material into theoretical products, such as taxonomies, key themes, or conceptual models. The remainder of the chapter will focus on these final two steps: analysis and theory development.

Developing Coding Schemes and Coding Data

Overview of Process

Codes are tags or labels for assigning units of meaning to descriptive or inferential information, and coding is the process of organizing the data into "chunks" that are alike, moving from words and sentence to "incidents," which are conceptually similar.[12,16] The process of coding takes place iteratively. Initial codes, including detailed operational definitions, are developed; these initial codes are applied to several units of analysis (e.g., transcripts, notes) and revised as needed to better encapsulate the data.

Developing Initial Coding Scheme

Codes are the building blocks of subsequent theory; therefore, developing the initial coding scheme is an essential part of moving from codes to theory. Approaches to developing the coding scheme vary, reflecting the diversity of analysis strategies. The first is the purely inductive, "grounded" approach.[11,13] This technique seeks to develop codes *de novo* based on concepts that emerge from the text without predetermined categories or guiding theory. Typically, the researchers begin by reviewing a small portion of the open-ended data and develop codes one by one as new concepts become apparent in the data. This process continues, with a re-reviewing of previously coded data as new codes are defined to ensure that the full properties of the codes have been captured. The coding scheme becomes larger and more detailed as more data are reviewed, until no new concepts are identified in the data. The final coding scheme developed by the end of the data review is then systematically reapplied to all transcripts to ensure all relevant data have been categorized.

A second approach is less "grounded" *per se* and involves researchers beginning with a provisional "start list"[12] of codes. The list of codes already has a clear structure and rationale, likely based on concepts and conceptual frameworks in the literature. Using this approach, researchers may identify general conceptual domains and codes *a priori* and then, within each domain, develop content-specific codes inductively.[20] For example, in a study of psychosocial factors related to long-term care financial planning,[21] the analysis was guided by Ajzen's theory of planned behavior.[22] The theory of planned behavior posits that attitudes, social norms and perceived control play a critical role in decision-making. Consistent with this theory, the analysis began with a broad list of codes, with these three domains initially representing the key psychosocial factors. Importantly, new domains such as individual rights and responsibilities were created as additional constructs emerged during analysis. In all approaches, the coding scheme should remain flexible, evolving as the iterative process of data collection and analysis continues.

Revising and Finalizing the Coding Scheme

Revisions to the initial coding scheme may include changes in definitions of codes, combining of two or more existing codes, and adding new codes or subcodes to represent emerging dimensions or properties of existing codes. New or different relationships among codes may be revealed, resulting in "bridging" or "extension" of codes.[17] As analysis continues, the operational definition of each code will become more precise with its properties more fully described. Coding typically employs the "constant comparative method"[11] of analysis, in which analysts constantly compare previously coded material to new material to refine codes and ensure conceptual homogeneity of each code. The process of refining and applying codes involves substantial and often lengthy negotiation among the team of analysts to define a final coding scheme. The final coding scheme, which is generally finalized only after review of all data, should include a list of all codes and their detailed definitions with examples of the types of data within each code. With this final code scheme, analysts then begin with the first transcript or observation again and apply the final coding scheme to all the data. Analysts may do this independently and check their reliability in coding formally[12,16] or may apply the final codes in a group, negotiating assigned codes through group discussion and consensus.

Types of Codes

Several types of codes are helpful to capture qualitative data and to facilitate subsequent analysis and theoretical products from the study. As shown in Table 1, the types of codes reflect: 1) the setting (e.g., place of care, type of practice); 2) characteristics of the participants (e.g., gender, insurance type, race/ethnicity, occupation, clinical discipline, geography of residence); 3) perspectives of the participant (e.g., positive, negative, non-committal); 4) conceptual domains or dimensions related to the phenomenon of interest (e.g., shared decision-making, quality of care, perceived control); and 5) relationships or patterns, which may be causal or non-causal, among concepts (e.g., a given factor may impede or encourage a particular behavior). Different types of codes are useful for different types of research questions and goals in theoretical development. Many studies, if coded comprehensively, draw upon all types of codes; however, studies need not employ all code types.

Table 1: Major Types of Codes for Qualitative Analysis

• The setting (e.g., place of care, type of practice)
• Characteristics of the participants (e.g., gender, insurance type, race/ethnicity, occupation, clinical discipline)
• Perspectives of the participant (e.g., positive, negative, non-committal)
• Conceptual domains or dimensions related to the phenomenon of interest (e.g., shared decision making, quality of care, perceived control)
• Relationships among concepts (e.g., a given factor may impede or encourage a particular behavior)

Codes that indicate the setting or participants' characteristics, termed "contextual codes" by some,[13] can facilitate theme comparisons across subgroups. For instance, one might compare data coded with a participant characteristic code such as "long-term care user" with the data coded with a participant characteristic code such as "long-term care non-user." Both the setting codes and the participant characteristic codes may be applied to full transcripts that are relevant, thus marking them for future subgroup analyses and comparisons.

Codes that indicate participants' perspectives help catalogue the direction of a viewpoint (e.g., is the participant favorable, unfavorable, or indifferent about the particular concept described). Such codes can be important for understanding not just the particular concept itself that may be described, but also what the participant thought or felt about the concept. As an example, in a study of individual's views on long-term care insurance, one might code statements about the difficulty finding accurate information about alternatives as a negative statement using a perspective code. Another statement indicating that long-term care insurance can improve access to needed home care services might be coded as a positive statement using a perspective code.

Codes that indicate concepts include both codes for conceptual domains and codes, or subcodes, for dimensions of those conceptual domains. Conceptual codes and subcodes (termed "axial coding" by others[13]) reflect what we term "vertical structure" in the coding scheme. They reflect structure in the sense that these codes encompass overarching concepts as well as the dimensions or axes that comprise the overarching concept. As an example,[23] the overarching conceptual might be "goals." The subcodes might be "content of the goal," "specificity of the goal," "challenge of the goal," and "sharedness of the goal." A future quantitative survey assessing goals, based on this taxonomy, would include items that measured the content, specificity, challenge, and sharedness of each goal. Unlike perspective codes, conceptual codes and subcodes are non-directional and indicate the concept itself, not whether the participant expressed positive or negative views concerning the concept, or whether there is a hypothesized relationship among codes.

The last code type is the relationship code. These codes are used to represent relationships among and between conceptual codes and hence reflect what we term the "horizontal structure" of the coding scheme. The codes may reflect a temporal sequence of actions (sometimes called "process" codes),[13,24] or they may reflect an inferred causal link among different conceptual categories or domains. The relationship codes reflect horizontal structure in the sense that the determinants (or temporally earlier processes, as relevant) typically appear graphically to the left of the consequences (or temporally later processes, as relevant) in the causal chain. For instance, in a study of health disparities[25] a patient's quotation stating that his/her negative experiences with physicians were a consequence of discriminatory treatment based on race was coded with a relationship code (e.g., "relationship of physician interactions and race"), suggesting the hypothesis that negative physician interactions are related to the patient's race.

Double Coding

Using these code types, analysts can apply two or more codes (also known as "code intersections") to a single incident, to tag the section of the transcript or observation as both a particular concept (i.e., quality of care) and a perspective (i.e., positive) to identify positive comments or views on quality of care. Further, the section might be further coded by the participant characteristic (i.e., long-term care user) to identify data illustrating positive views of long-term care among long-term care users. In this way, detailed coding can facilitate more specific analyses, especially comparative analyses across subgroups by setting or participant characteristics.

Linking Codes to Theory

The theoretical products from qualitative research may include one or more of the following: a taxonomy or classification system of a complex phenomenon, a set of key themes, or a conceptual model. The process from moving from the coded data to the theory differs based on the intended product of the analysis. The output may stand alone as a theoretical contribution to the literature or may be used to prompt further research, sometimes with larger samples and quantitative methodology to complement the qualitative, theoretical work.

Developing Taxonomy

Taxonomies are classification systems of complex, multifaceted phenomena, which articulate the dimensions or axes of the larger phenomenon. Taxonomies contribute to the theoretical and descriptive literature about multifaceted phenomenon, programs, and interventions. In addition, they are useful as a foundation for developing subsequent measurement instruments, which may be used in quantitative research. Whereas the taxonomy articulates the various aspects of some phenomenon, a survey instrument with specific items designed to tap the concepts from the taxonomy can ensure more accurate measurement. Such accurate measurement is critical for valid and reliable evaluation of multifaceted programs or interventions. Examples of taxonomies have been developed across a broad array of clinical and health services research areas.[23,26-28]

Taxonomies are developed primarily from the data tagged with conceptual codes and their subcodes, or what we termed the "vertical structure." Using the larger conceptual domain codes, the major aspects or axes of the phenomenon of interest can be defined and described; data tagged by conceptual subcodes can then further refine each domain into its key dimensions. Depending on the scope of the phenomenon, the dimensions may be characterized at an additional level, reflecting their primary properties.

For example, in a taxonomy classifying quality improvement, which is a broad and multifaceted term potentially encompassing many concepts and aspects, we define six domains that comprise quality improvement efforts in the hospital setting: organizational goals, administrative support, clinician leadership, performance improvement initiatives, use of data, and contextual factors. Dimensions for each of the domains are then also specified, with exemplar concepts or ranges of each dimension. See Figure 1 for a display of this taxonomy. Note that each domain was represented in the coding as a conceptual code, and the dimensions were represented by subcodes within each of those domains.

Themes can be developed from coded qualitative data in a variety of ways. These include the use of explicit statements to develop themes, employing implicit interpretation to develop themes, and conducting comparative analyses to develop themes. No single approach is stronger than another; rather the recommended approach depends on the research question and scope of data available for analysis.

Explicit statements. First, themes can be developed based on explicit statements by participants about what they see as determinants or consequences of the phenomenon of interest. Ideally, these explicit statements are coded with relationship codes and easily summarized to reflect participants' perceptions of various causal connections among the coded

Factors/Dimensions	Concepts
Goals	
Content	Improve patient care; maintain financial position; enhance reputation
Specificity	Explicit performance targets set vs more vague goal of improving generally
Challenge	Zero-defects vs more lenient goals
Sharedness	Widespread sharing of and agreement with goal vs conflicting/unsupported goals
Administrative support	
Philosophy	Supportive of quality improvement; indifferent; negative
Resources	Human technical resource availability; training in quality improvement techniques
Clinical support	
Physician, nurse, and ancillary clinical staff leadership and support	Presence and participation of leaders/facilitators and/or detractors from improvement efforts
PI initiatives	
Initiative type	Enhancing adherence to existing system; redesigning existing system
Implementation style	Participation vs autocracy; focus on improvement vs fault-finding; methods used to increase adherence to standards; consequences of compliance or non-compliance; degree of teamwork
Use of data	
Validity	Source and perceived quality of the data
Timeliness	Report frequency; reflecting recent practice
Benchmarking	Use of data from comparable sites, groups, or physician peers to aid in interpretation of hospital or physician performance
Modifying factors	
Hospital size	Capacity; staffed beds
System affiliation	Part of health system vs independent
Ownership type	Non-profit; for-profit; government-owned
Financial constraints	Degree of competition for cardiac care
Organizational turbulence	Turnover of senior administrative/clinical staff; mergers/acquisitions; unionization

PI = performance improvement

Figure 1: Taxonomy of Quality Improvement Efforts

Source: Bradley E.H., et al. Qualitative Study of Increasing Beta-Blocker use After Myocardial Infarction: Why do Some Hospitals Succeed? *JAMA,* 2001; 285:2604-2611.

concepts. The richness of these data depends on the data collection approach and the degree to which "why" questions were asked and answered during interviews or observations with participants. Individual participants may be constrained in their ability to hypothesize about the causal connections, as participants are influenced by their role in the experience and are unlikely to have access to the full range of participants' experiences.

Implicit interpretation. A second approach to developing themes or hypotheses draws on the implicit interpretation by the researcher of the participants' statements. A researcher may hypothesize that one concept is associated with or causes another event based on how the stories are told, including the sequence of events. Using this approach, the themes and hypotheses are based on the researcher's analysis of what appears to be conceptually linked.

Comparative analyses. A third approach, which also uses implicit interpretation of participants' statements, identifies patterns and potentially causal connections by performing comparative analyses by subgroup. In this approach, data coded within the conceptual codes are separated according to the setting or the characteristics of the participants to compare whether the concepts described in one group differ qualitatively from those described in a comparison group. The comparison can be performed using formal comparative methods[29] or using more qualitative inspection of perspectives or concepts that may be described differently in comparison groups. Examples of key theme development[1,25,30-32] using explicit statements by participants, using implicit analysis, and using formal comparative analysis again are represented in a diverse range of clinical and health services research. One example from the public health literature is a study examining socioeconomic status and dissatisfaction with the health care system among chronically ill African Americans.[30] In-depth interviews with chronically ill African Americans were used to elicit experiences and perceptions regarding the health care system. Transcripts were analyzed using the constant comparative method to identify central emergent themes from the data. Recurrent themes addressed socioeconomic status and perceptions of health care, dissatisfaction with care among low income persons, questioning of whether discrimination is present, and changes in health care coverage.

Developing Conceptual Models

A conceptual model represents a set of propositions or a set of hypotheses concerning the relationships between various determinants, mediating factors, and consequences of the phenomena of interest. Therefore, techniques for developing conceptual models are similar to the approaches for developing themes or hypotheses. However, conceptual models and theories comprise multiple hypotheses and relationships, and thus the analysis becomes more expansive and complex as the number of possible relationships grows. Examples of using qualitative research to develop conceptual models or theory are most common in the nursing literature but are also apparent in clinical and health services research fields.[33-35]

In the field of gerontology, for example, the expanded Andersen model[33] of long-term care use is a conceptual model developed from qualitative research. The model is intended to generate comprehensive identification of psychosocial factors to improve understanding of the complex relationships between race/ethnicity and long-term care use, as well as to inform development of programs and policies designed to address disparities in long term care use among minority and non-minority groups. The model was developed using a "start list" of overarching codes, reflecting Andersen's behavioral health services use model,[36] for predisposing, need, and enabling factors. Focus group data were then tagged with both conceptual codes to illuminate the additional boxes shown in the model in Figure 2 (i.e., attitudes toward services, social norms about caregiving, and perceived control) as well as relationship codes to provide evidence for the lines that connect the boxes in the model in Figure 2. Each line represents a hypothesis, which is supported by explicit statements of participants. As described above, hypothesized causal connections can also be developed through researchers' inferences based on implicit statements or by researchers' comparative analyses of statements by subgroups.

Enhancing the Process of Moving from Codes to Theory

Experts in qualitative methods[12,15,37-38] have suggested a number of strategies for ensuring the overall quality and rigor of qualitative research. Some of these strategies are particularly germane to the process of moving from the codes to the theory. We recommend using multiple researchers with differing disciplines in the process of developing coding schemes, applying codes, and developing theory from the coded data. A multidisciplinary research team allows for group discussions and negotiation concerning the meaning of unclear or subjective data, which in turn can enhance the breadth and understanding of qualitative data. Additionally, we recommend using participant validation of the theory to the extent feasible. Allowing a subset of participants to read the theory for face validity can be helpful. Third, we suggest consistent application of the coding scheme to all transcripts or observations, once the coding scheme has been finalized. Last, given the complexity of the process of theoretical development, we recommend the

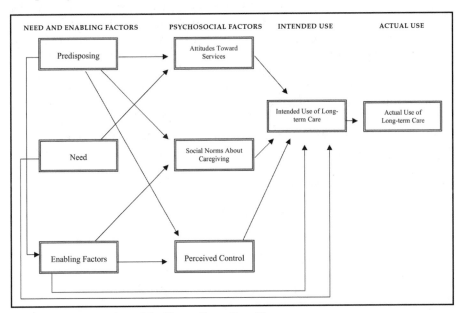

Figure 2: Conceptual Model of Long-Term Care Use

Source: Bradley E.H. et al., Expanding the Andersen Model: the Role of Psychosocial Factors in Long-Term Care Use. *Health Services Research,* 2002; 37:1221-1242.

maintenance of a detailed audit trail, which might include memos about insights at different points in the process, the regularly updated coding schemes with definitions and properties described, and analytic decisions made through the process. With these efforts, the creative process by which taxonomies, key themes, and conceptual models "emerge" from coded data becomes more explicit and replicable, potentially leading to more valuable and credible insights from qualitative work.

Conclusions

Theoretical products from qualitative research include, but are not limited to, taxonomies, key themes, and conceptual models. While each of these contributes to theory development itself, they also have practical applications. Taxonomies are used to improve the measurement and thus the accurate comparison and evaluation of complex, multifaceted interventions, which are commonplace in clinical, health services, and health policy research and practice. Themes and hypotheses can provide practical information about nuances of interventions, which can help refine and increase the effectiveness of programs and policies. Conceptual models can guide future empirical work to ensure that the questions we ask quantitatively are grounded in sensible and realistic models of behavior and practice.

Codes types include setting, characteristics of participants, participant perspectives, conceptual domains and dimensions, and relationship codes. Taxonomy development draws on data tagged with conceptual domains and dimension codes. Themes and hypotheses, as well as conceptual model development, draw on data tagged with conceptual codes and relationship codes. The quality of the analytical process of moving from codes to theory benefits from multiple coders and analysts, consistent development and use of a coding scheme, and comprehensive audit trails to document analytic decisions.

Theory development is a slow and laborious process, which can be facilitated through deliberate coding of data and particular attention to setting, participant characteristics, perspectives, conceptual domains and dimensions, and relationships among codes. There has previously been limited guidance regarding specific techniques of moving from the codes to the theory in qualitative research. We propose a set of theoretical products as well as coding and analytical approaches to generate those products.

Summary Points
- Qualitative research is ideal for producing taxonomies of complex phenomena, themes or hypotheses, and conceptual frameworks.
- Code types include setting, characteristics of participants, participant perspectives, conceptual domains and dimensions, and relationship codes.
- Taxonomy development draws on data tagged with conceptual domains and dimension codes.
- Themes and hypotheses, as well as conceptual model development, draw on data tagged with conceptual codes and relationship codes.
- The quality of the analytical process of moving from codes to theory benefits from multiple coders and analysts, consistent development and use of a coding scheme, and comprehensive audit trails to document analytic decisions.

References

1) Marshall, M.N., Mannion. R., Nelson, E., and Davies, H.T. Managing Change in the Culture of General Practice: Qualitative Case Studies in Primary Care Trusts. *BMJ.* 2003; 327: 599-602.

2) Craigie, F.C. Jr. and Hobbs, F.R. Exploring the Organizational Culture of Exemplary Community Health Center Practices. *Family Medicine.* 2004;36:733-8.

3) Marshall, M.N. Improving Quality in General Practice: Qualitative Case Study of Barriers Faced by Health Authorities. *BMJ.* 1999; 319:164-7

4) Donovan, J. et al. Quality Improvement Report: Improving Design and Conduct of Randomised Trials by Embedding Them in Qualitative Research: ProtecT (prostate Testing for Cancer and Treatment) Study. *BMJ* 2002; 325:766-70.

5) Bradley, E.H. et al. Translating Research into Practice: Making Change Happen. *Journal of American Geriatrics Society.* 2004; 52:1875-1882.

6) Koops, L. and Lindley, R.I. Thrombolysis for Acute Ischaemic Stroke: Consumer Involvement in Design of New Randomised Controlled Trial. *BMJ.* 2002; 415-417.

7) Stapleton, H., Kirkham, M., and Thomas, G. Qualitative Study of Evidence Based Leaflets in Maternity Care. *BMJ.* 2002; 324:639-643.

8) Mays, N. and Pope, C. Rigour and Qualitative Research. *BMJ.* 1995;311:109-12.

9) Pope, C. and Mays, N. Reaching the Parts Other Methods Cannot Reach: An Introduction to Qualitative Methods in Health and Health Services Research. *BMJ.* 1995;311:42-5.

10) Giacomini, M.K. and Cook, D.J. Users' Guides to the Medical Literature: XXIII. Qualitative Research in Health Care A. Are the Results of the Study Valid? Evidence-Based Medicine Working Group. *JAMA.* 2000;284:357-62.

11) Glaser, B.G. and Strauss, A.L. *The Discovery of Grounded Theory: Strategies for Qualitative Research.* New York: Aldine De Gruyter, 1967.

12) Miles, M,B. and Huberman, A.M. *Qualitative Data Analysis: A Sourcebook of New Methods* (2nd ed.). Beverly Hills: Sage Publications, 1994.

13) Strauss, A. and Corbin, J. *Basics of Qualitative Research.* Thousand Oaks, CA: Sage Publications, 1998.

14) Crabtree, B. and Miller, W. *Doing Qualitative Research,* (2nd Ed.). Newbury Park, CA: Sage, 1999.

15) Patton, M.Q. *Qualitative Research and Evaluation Methods* (3rd ed.). Thousand Oaks, CA: Sage Publications. 2002.

16) Boyatzis, R. *Transforming Qualitative Information: Thematic Analysis and Code Development.* Thousand Oaks, CA: Sage, 1998.

17) Lincoln, Y.S. and Guba, E.G. *Naturalistic Inquiry.* Beverly Hills CA: Sage, 1985.

18) Creswell, J.W. *Research Design: Qualitative, Quantitative, and Mixed Methods Approaches.* Thousand Oaks, CA: Sage Publications, 2003.

19) Pope, C., Ziebland, S., and Mays, N. Qualitative Research in Health Care. Analysing Qualitative Data. *BMJ.* 2000; 320:114-116.

20) Lofland, J. *Analyzing Social Settings: A Guide to Qualitative Observation and Analysis.* Belmont, CA: Wadsworth, 1971.

21) Curry, L.A., Bradley, E.H., and Robison, J. Individual Decisions in Financing Nursing Home Care: Psychosocial Considerations, *Journal of Aging Studies,* 2004; 18: 337-352.

22) Ajzen, I. From Intentions to Actions: A Theory of Planned Behavior. In K. Kuhland, and J. Beckman (Eds.). *Action-Control: From Cognitions to Behavior.* Heidelberg: Springer, 1985, pp. 11-39.

23) Bogardus, S.T., Bradley, E.H., Inouye, S.K., and Tinetti, M. A Taxonomy for Goal Setting in the Care of Persons with Dementia. *Journal of General Internal Medicine.* 1998; 13:675-680.

24) Bogden, R. and Biklen, S.K. *Qualitative Research for Education: An Introduction to Theory and Methods* (2nd Edition). Boston: Allyn and Bacon, 1992.

25) Bates, M.S., Rankin-Hill, L. and Sanchez, Ayendez M. The Effects of the Cultural Context of Health Care on Treatment of and Response to Chronic Pain and Illness. *Social Science and Medicine.* 1997; 45:1433-1447.

26) Porter, E.J., Ganong, L.H., Drew, N., and Lanes, T.I. A New Typology of Home-Care Helpers. *Gerontologist.* 2004;44:750-9

27) Ely, J.W. et al. Obstacles to Answering Doctors' Questions about Patient Care with Evidence: Qualitative Study. *BMJ.* 2002; 324(7339):710-716.

28) Bradley, E.H., et al. A Qualitative Study of Increasing Beta-Blocker use After Myocardial Infarction: Why do Some Hospitals Succeed? *JAMA.* 2001; 285:2604-2611.

29) Ragin, C.C. *The Comparative Method: Moving Beyond Qualitative and Quantitative Strategies.* Los Angeles, CA: University of California Press, 1987.

30) Becker, G., Gates, R.J. and Newsom, E. Self-Care Among Chronically Ill African Americans: Culture, Health Disparities, and Health Insurance Status *Am J Public Health.* 2004; 94:2066–2073

31) Gallagher, T.H. et al. Patients and Physicians' Attitudes Regarding the Disclosure of Medical Errors. *JAMA* 2003; 289:1001-1007

32) Benson, J. and Britten, N. Patients' Decisions About Whether or Not to Take Antihypertensive Drugs: Qualitative Study. *BMJ.* 2002;325:873-878

33) Bradley E.H. et al. Expanding the Andersen Model: The Role of Psychosocial Factors in Long-Term Care Use. *Health Services Research.* 2002; 37:1221-1242.

34) Davidson, P.L., Andersen, R.M., Wyn, R., and Brown, E.R. A Framework for Evaluating Safety-Net and Other Community-Level Factors on Access for Low-Income Populations. *Inquiry.* 2004;41:21-38.

35) Martin, D.K., Thiel, E.C., and Singer, P.A. A New Model of Advance Care Planning: Observations from People with HIV. *Archives of Internal Medicine.* 1999;159:86-92

36) Andersen, R.M. Revisiting the Behavioral Model and Access to Medical Care: Does it Matter? *Journal of Health and Social Behavior.* 1995; 36:1-10.

37) Mays, N. and Pope, C. Assessing Quality in Qualitative Research. *BMJ.* 2000; 320:50-52.

38) Kirk, J. and Miller, M. Reliability and Validity in Qualitative Research. *Qualitative Research Method Series,* Vol. 1.475. London: Sage, 1986.

Chapter 9

Preserving Cultural Integrity through Analysis

Yewoubdar Beyene, PhD

Introduction

Qualitative methods have become common in research that addresses the social and cultural dimensions of health and illness.[1,2] Qualitative researchers draw upon and utilize the approaches, methods, and techniques of ethnography, participant observation, phenomenology, hermeneutics, psychoanalysis, cultural studies, survey research, and ecological studies among others.[3] These methods derive from several social science disciplines, and the concepts, knowledge and methods of each disciplinary tradition vary. Qualitative research design depends on the study matter in question, and the kinds of questions that are asked depend on their context.

In this chapter we describe the potential contribution of anthropological research methods in health studies. We use examples from Mexico, Greece, and Cameroon as a way to highlight differences and similarities in perceptions and practices about health behaviors and aging. By improving our understanding of the relativity of health practices and attitudes in the world through the use of rigorous comparison, we are better able to enhance our appreciation of health practices and attitudes in the United States.

The Anthropological Contribution

Anthropology has a vast cross-cultural literature that is a vibrant source of comparison, ideas, and tools for general understanding of the human condition. Anthropologists adopt a highly elastic approach and draw upon many methods of data collection and analysis in order to achieve a fuller understanding of a particular phenomenon. As a result, anthropology in general does not lend itself to the stark division between qualitative and quantitative methods.[5] Therefore, it is as appropriate to collect quantitative data (e.g., demographic data, household economic data, prevalence of illness, disease, attitudes), as it is to collect qualitative data through cultural immersion.[5,6]

With its multiple emphases on biological, cultural, ecological, linguistic, and historical factors, anthropology has a unique contribution to make to our understanding of health and illness.[4,5] The research methods of anthropology may be different from those of other disciplines that use qualitative methods, because they are always comparative and holistic.[6] The holistic research approach in anthropology refers to the efforts to integrate various levels of analysis from the biological to the cultural; the present and the past; and the local and the global that allows anthropologists to see the big picture. This orientation sets anthropological research apart from other disciplines. The underlying premise of this approach is that the whole system must be understood in its complexity to understand any part in isolation.[5,6]

Anthropology has a theoretical and methodological history with a distinctive approach to gathering and analyzing data that can yield productive insights into the subject under study by examining the study topic within its broader social and cultural contexts.[5,6] A core conceptual feature of anthropology is that it defines what is rational within a broader cultural context.

Anthropology has made important methodological contributions to public health[7,8] and to studies of health and aging.[9–11] The use of systematic descriptive qualitative methods has proven effective in identifying context-specific factors that contribute to health. The salience of this view for understanding issues in health care is vital. The holistic approach is distinct to the discipline and offers relevant conceptual frameworks, substantive knowledge, and methodological insights by integrating the various aspects of health and disease. Another significant methodological contribution of anthropology to health and aging is in the use of triangulation, by systematically applying multiple methods in order to reduce bias in situations where controlled comparison is not feasible.[12]

The following outline highlights the main characteristics of anthropological approach such as the role of the interviewer in qualitative study; principals of participant-observation and comparative methods and two case examples from my work that illustrate holistic and integrative data analysis in anthropology.

The Role of the Interviewer

The interviewer in qualitative research is the key to the quality of data gathering and data analysis. Unlike quantitative data analysis, qualitative data analysis requires that the researcher has first-hand knowledge of the research setting, the culture under study, and the data that have been collected.[13,14] The quality of data obtained in qualitative study can vary considerably depending upon the skills of the interviewer in establishing rapport, following up leads, and demonstrating attention and interest. In qualitative data collection, the role of the interviewer is very critical. One has to be aware that the interview is influenced by the identities and roles of the researcher.[15] Very often the interviewer does not always choose nor control her/his roles and identities in the field, but learns to follow roles imposed by others or negotiated in the research setting.[13] Furthermore, the personal characteristics of the interviewer have a major impact on rapport, the set of questions which the interviewer is socially allowed to ask, and the responses with which he/she empathizes. For example, if an interviewer is intolerant about premarital sex, one should not expect the interviews to contain much material on that topic, both because the interviewer is uncomfortable pursuing the idea and because the respondent may sense the interviewer's judgmental attitude. It is thus essential that the person analyzing the transcript and output knows something about the personal characteristics of the interviewer and takes these considerations into account.

Effective interviewing is a complex task requiring attendance to a range of skills and information at the same time and requires rigorous training to minimize interview bias. The requirement of immersion in the culture under study through participant observation, and keeping of detailed field notes and a personal diary of one's experience in the field, have been very useful in minimizing interviewer bias in anthropological study.[13,16] In contrast to survey data, anthropological qualitative data are easier to take these influences into account during analysis because they may be readily detectable from both the interview transcript and any accompanying observational notes made about the respondent and the interaction.

Participant Observation

Participant observation is anthropology's most characteristic research strategy, which involves direct observation while participating in the study community.[16] A key anthropological contribution to health and aging research lies in its empirically-based grasp of the context-specific nature of social processes. This focus on the particular, which anthropology insists on through documenting the complex details of everyday life, provides an important corrective to generalizations and abstractions that can often mislead.[17] What people say they do, and what they actually do are often very different. Therefore, what people do, including how and why they do it, are important aspects of qualitative data and should be integrated in the analysis. These questions are substantiated not only qualitatively through interview data and narrative analysis, but also from observational data that might be descriptive or quantitative in nature. Documenting the observable data such as routines of everyday life, physical settings (where people live, work, etc.), and describing expressed emotions (anger, sadness, laughter, eye contact or lack of, etc.) during interviews are essential components in qualitative research that should be an integral part of the data analysis.

Comparative Analysis

The term "comparative" in anthropology refers to paying attention to diversity when trying to learn about a particular phenomenon and then attempting to generalize from the information obtained.[5] Comparison is essential to anthropological research. To understand cultural factors, societies must be compared. Data analysis in anthropology involves sifting and sorting through pieces of data to detect and interpret thematic categorizations, searching for inconsistencies and contradictions, and generating conclusions about what is happening and why. Comparing primary data with secondary sources can produce strong results. For example, comparing interviews to archival data on an issue of symptom reporting and response in different settings can produce stronger analytical insights with greater potential generalizability. This is achieved through logical, rather than statistical, inferences that make use of relevant empirical knowledge and theoretical principles.[18]

The remaining sections of this chapter elaborate on the methodological approaches of anthropology and focus on medical anthropology and the use of biocultural analysis in the study of social, cultural, and biological dimensions of health and aging. Biocultural analysis provides insight by synthesizing the interplay among cultural, ecological, and biological forces in health and illness.[4,6]

Comparative Methods and Data Analysis in Reproductive Aging Study

The following two studies illustrate principles of and approaches to integrative analysis of cultural, biological, and ecological data in a qualitative anthropological study. The study of cross-cultural health practices highlights how these complex factors interact as well as how various societies exhibit contrasting health behaviors and expectations. The first example illustrates the use of comparative methods in a study of reproductive aging. The second example illustrates the integration of qualitative and quantitative data sources in a public health related study.

Cross-Cultural Comparison of Menopausal Experiences of Women
Cross-cultural studies of menopause question the assumption of the biological universality of women's experiences.[19-22] Assumptions about the existence of a universal, "natural" menstrual history have been refuted by anthropological evidence, which indicates considerable cross-cultural variation in all aspects of menstrual cycling.[23] Since all meaning is culturally specific, the cultural meanings of menopause may vary from place to place. At the same time, menopause is also part of the physiological history of most women's reproductive lives. Attempts to make a distinction between the menopausal experiences of women based on social and cultural factors alone may give rise to misleading conclusions.[19] If menopause is principally a hormonal event, one would expect that women throughout the world would experience symptoms in the same way. Since menopause is part of a woman's reproductive life, it should be examined within the context of the reproductive history of a woman, which is linked to social, cultural, and ecological variables.

The data presented below were obtained from an extended ethnographic study that investigated and compared the natural history of the menopausal experiences of women in subsistence farming communities in two cultures. The cultures studied were rural Mayan Indians in Yucatan, Mexico, and rural Greek women living on the island of Evia (Euboea), Greece[19].

The data were collected using a systematic ethnographic approach and consisted of the following sources: census taking; intensive participant-observation; unstructured interviews with key informants (including midwives, older and younger women, traditional healers, physicians, and medical personnel in the health services and clinics that served the area); and life history interviews of pre-menopausal, menopausal, and postmenopausal women. These extensive interviews gathered demographic and reproductive data, data on women's general health, and women's experiences of and attitudes toward menstruation and menopause, diet, and daily activities.

Similarities and contrasts among the two groups. The data from Mayan and Greek women indicated some similarities as well as marked differences between women in the two cultures. While the women seemed to share similar cultural values with respect to beliefs and practices regarding menstruation and child bearing, roles of women, attitudes toward aging, they differed in their experiences with menopause, childbearing patterns, diet, and the ecological niche in which they lived.

Both Mayan and Greek women regarded menopause as a natural phenomenon that all women experience. Both groups of women emphasized the relief and freedom that menopause offers from unwanted pregnancy and the cultural taboos associated with menstruation. However, the Mayan and Greek women in the study differed in their fertility history, the age for onset of menopause, the experience of menopausal symptoms, and diet, which is linked to the ecological habitat of each group.

Mayan women married in their teens, some as early as 13–14 years of age, had numerous pregnancies, did not use contraceptive methods, breastfed their children on an average of two years, had lactation amenorrhea of 18–24 months, and sometimes reported having few or no periods between pregnancies. The onset of menopause among Mayan women was relatively early: the average age for onset of menopause was 42, and a large number of women experienced menopause in their thirties. Menopausal symptoms, other than the session of menses, were not culturally recognized. None of the women interviewed reported hot flashes. The Mayan diet is high in carbohydrates and low in animal protein due to ecological and socio-political variables.

The Greek women in the study married in their mid-twenties, reported common use of contraceptives such as condoms, on average had 2–3 pregnancies, and breastfed for only 6-9 months. The average age for onset of menopause was 47 (with a large number congregated between the ages of 45-55). Menopausal symptoms such as hot flashes and cold sweats were culturally recognized, and both menopausal and postmenopausal women reported experiencing hot flashes. Greek women considered menopausal symptoms a temporary discomfort rather than a symptom of illness. Whereas these women use a variety of herbal remedies to alleviate menstrual discomfort, they did not use herbal remedies nor seek medical help for menopausal symptom relief. Greek women had varied dietary resources that consisted of grains and a good deal of animal protein.

This comparison suggests that the perception of and experience of menopause vary cross-culturally. However, the comparison also suggests that the presence or absence of physiological symptoms cannot be accounted for simply by role changes at middle age or by the affects of cultural taboos. The roles of culture and biology constitute women's experiences, and expressions of menopause are often intertwined in complicated ways. Thus, the lack of physiological symptoms such as hot flashes among the Mayan women and almost a decade difference in age for onset of menopause between Greek and Mayan women calls for explanation beyond social and cultural factors alone. Menopause is part of a woman's reproductive process and the age for onset of menopause and hot flashes are phenomena induced by hormonal changes.[24,25] Therefore, the analysis in this study had to integrate the various cultural and biological factors that affect reproductive hormone production. In doing so, the study suggests that the diet and fertility patterns may affect both the timing of menopause as well as how menopause is experienced.

It has been documented that nutrition plays a role in reproduction, and differences in hormone production between populations have been partly accounted for by differences in diet. Caloric restriction decreases the age of natural menopause.[26] Interrelated factors, such as under-nutrition, in conjunction with the demands of menstruation, pregnancy, lactation and heavy daily work load with high energy expenditure, can lead to premature aging of women.[27] Therefore, the study concluded that diet and fertility patterns could be accounted for the differences in menopausal age and experiences of Mayan and Greek women in the study.

The Importance of Biological as Well as Cultural Factors in Analysis

By comparing the reproductive histories of women from two different societies, it is therefore possible to isolate historical, cultural, and environmental factors that relate to variations or similarities in response to menopause. Some studies based solely on biomedical assumptions neglect how women in non-industrialized, traditional societies have different fertility patterns than women in Western industrialized societies. These patterns, in turn, may expose them to different levels of reproductive hormones, including estrogen. The results from this comparative study provide a dramatic demonstration that the reproductive process of menopause, like other human developmental phases, is shaped by the cultural, ecological, and social environments of women.

Moreover, data from this comparative study provided a base for a multidisciplinary research project that examined the relationship of early menopause and bone density among Mayan women in Yucatan.[20] The ethnographic data showed that Mayan women have a high calcium and low protein diet, maintain a relatively high level of physical activity, are relatively obese, and do not smoke or drink alcohol. None of the elderly women report a history of bone fracture.

The absence of hot flashes and apparent protection from fracture raised the question of whether the menopausal transition is endocrinologically different among Mayan women. We pursued this line of inquiry using quantitative and qualitative methods that included: a survey of the prevalence of fracture in the population from clinical reports, hospital records, individual fracture histories; medical and reproductive histories; physical activity and dietary calcium assessments; physical examinations including height and weight, blood pressures; brief cardiopulmonary examinations; and blood samples for hormonal concentration assessments and radial bone density assessment (for more detail on this study see Beyene and Martin[20]). (See also work by Del Vecchio, Good, et al. on more examples of comparative studies[28,29]).

Integrating Interviews, Archival, and Ecological Data in a Qualitative Public Health Study

The following study illustrates the benefits of combining methods in order to better understand a health-related topic. Using data from focus groups, individual key informant interviews, participant-observation and four years of birth records from two main hospitals in the area, this research explored the relationship among maternal workloads, seasonality of birth, availability of food, and patterns of lactation among the Nso women of North West Cameroon.[34]

Breast-Feeding Patterns and Women's Work in North West Cameroon

In the 1990s, most developing countries were instructed to adopt the Innocenti Declaration.[30] This initiative declared as a global goal for optimal maternal and child health and nutrition that all women should breast-feed, and that infants should be fed exclusively on breast milk from birth to 4–6 months of age. It further stipulated that breast-feeding should continue for up to two years while receiving supplemental food. There are two major reasons for encouraging women in developing countries to breast-feed their children. First, by reducing the use of unclean water in powdered milk, breast-feeding decreases the chances of infant diarrheal disease; and second, breast-feeding is generally associated with a period of infertility and prolonged interbirth intervals.[31–33]

The adoption of the WHO initiative of nonsupplemented breast-feeding has been challenging in sub-Saharan Africa where women do most of the agricultural work, and an overwhelming majority of women supplement their breast milk with gruel, often from the first weeks or even the first day of the baby's life. Maternal and child health and nutrition policies appear to focus on the child's well-being and overlook the various ecological, cultural, and social factors affecting breast-feeding and mothers' health.

Focus groups, interviews, and observations. The purpose of the focus group discussions was to obtain general contextual information on the cultural norms and issues affecting breast-feeding practices. Focus group participants ranged in age from 17–96 years old. We conducted nineteen focus group discussions with 6–9 women in each group.

Analysis of the data from the focus groups and key informant interviews showed that breast-feeding is a cultural norm in the North West Province of Cameroon. All women in the study group reported having breast-fed their children. However, the time for completely weaning children from breast milk varied by generation. The older group of women breast-fed their children from two to three years; the younger generation reported having breast-fed for only 1–1½ (one – one half years). All women stated that they gave their children "pap," thin corn gruel one to three months after birth. Women begin supplementing breast-feeding at various times, as early as the first week or as late as six months after birth. The baby's needs and the mother's milk supply determined the time of introduction of such foods. Because male infants are considered heavy feeders and female infants light feeders, mothers supplemented breast milk with gruel earlier for boys than for girls.

Moreover, the interview data also suggested inconsistencies in the pattern and timing of supplemental breast-feeding each time a woman gave birth, regardless of the gender of the baby. For example, a woman with five children would have a varied timeline of supplementing her breast-feeding for each child. The main reason given by the women for supplementing their baby's diet with solid food was their low milk production. Furthermore, data from participant-observation indicated that babies always slept with their mothers, are kept close to their mothers, and are carried on their backs. All farming women took their babies with them to farm and work a full day tilling the land, planting, weeding, and harvesting. They brought "pap" with them to supplement breast milk.

While the interview and observational data explained the patterns and cultural norms of breast-feeding, they did not explain why women reported varied patterns of breast milk production. Cultural norms are usually taken for granted by members of a society, and as a result, interviews about cultural behaviors do not always elicit the reasons why people do what they do. Therefore, researchers must sift through the available data in order to provide insight into the possible factors that may impact, for example, a woman's milk production. Because reproductive issues such as breast-feeding are influenced by biological and cultural factors,[24] the reasons for low milk production among farming women should therefore be looked at within the context of their lives.

By combining interview data with data from participant-observation, daily work patterns, and birth records, we attempted to find out why women's patterns of breast-feeding supplementation and milk production varied among farming women in North West Cameroon. This kind of triangulation of data sources in our analysis assisted us in identifying the factors that affected breast milk production. These factors included women's work patterns, seasonality of access to food, and seasonality of birth rates, which were all related to the ecological and cultural environments and to the role of women in the region.

Women's workloads: As throughout West Africa,[35] women in North West Cameroon are the main producers of food, and tilling the land, planting, weeding, and harvesting are the responsibilities of women. Women's time is usually fully taken up by a multitude of domestic and production tasks, and they spend considerable time walking to complete their daily tasks. Women also perform heavy work in terms of head-loading produce to market and in carrying water, fuel wood, and consumer goods.

Women's caloric intake: Although women said that they take food with them to the farm, it appears that the poor nutritional and caloric value of the food may be insufficient for producing milk as well as for working the land. Mostly, they take "fufu" corn porridge with "jama jama" green leafy vegetables cooked in palm oil. Data from interviews and participant observation indicate that the availability and consumption of food decrease during intense farm work season. The nutritional intake may not be adequate to sustain the high-energy requirement of a physically strenuous way of life as well as the demands of lactation.

Availability of food: Availability of foods and fruits is seasonal in nature. In agricultural societies such as rural Cameroon where there is one main crop a year, food is freely available after the harvest, but with storage losses and use, there may be little left in the growing season prior to the next harvest.[35] Potatoes and ground nuts (peanuts), corn, and beans, the main stable food, are available from June to October. Food availability starts to decrease at the end of October. March, April, and May are low food seasons and are also a time of intense work for women. In June, food availability starts to improve significantly, and agricultural activities start to decrease.

Agricultural activities require a high level of energy expenditure. Overall, energy expenditure of women in rural African communities is considered to be higher than that of men.[36] Since agricultural activities tend to be seasonal, the overall energy expenditure of women tends to vary with the season. It is higher during the rainy season and relatively low during the dry season. In this regard, season has been identified as one of the factors influencing the level of energy expenditure, and therefore, the nutritional status of rural African subsistence farm women.[37] During the rainy season the volume of activities increases and this coincides with the period of low food stocks, higher food prices, and low food intake. The quantity as well as the quality of foods available is directly affected by the season. For those women who are breastfeeding during the time of intense work season, the undernourished mother has a lower yield of milk, and the requirements for infant feeding may not be fully met.

Seasonality of birth: Pregnancy requires the availability of sufficient calories, and the timing of pregnancy appears to correlate with the seasons in which women have less work and more available foods. Therefore, local hospitals' birth record data indicated that most women became pregnant in the months (June, July, and September) when food is in abundance and workloads are low. They gave birth during the months (March, April, and May) of high work demands and low availability of food, which strongly affects their breast milk production capacity.

Among the Nso women, breast milk remains a vital element of the infants' diet for several years. Because of this length of time the chances that lactation coincides with the agricultural labor peak and low food availability seasons are greater. Therefore the fluctuating caloric conditions during this extended time have considerable impact on a woman's nutritional and health status during lactation as well as on her ability to produce enough breast milk to feed a baby without supplementation.[33,38] Lactation represents a higher relative metabolic load for poorly nourished mothers with high workload demands than for well-nourished mothers or mothers with low workloads. Policies on maternal and child health and nutrition should therefore take the workload demands and lactational metabolic load of farming women into consideration.

Conclusion

The cross-cultural examples from the studies discussed above provide compelling evidence that health practices and attitudes about aging are varied and complex throughout the world. Furthermore, the study design and data collection methods described in these studies are all within the scope of anthropological inquiry and illustrate the wide range of data sources as well as the strength of each data source to form a culturally integrated explanation of the study topic. The strength of such an approach is that relying on multiple data sources reduces the probability of drawing erroneous conclusions.[1,2,5,12] Where inconsistencies among the reported data existed, explanations were sought from the various data sources.

The menopause study demonstrates how comparative methods use data from various circumstances which are then integrated to infer how people deal with life events such as menopause.

Both studies show not only the advantages of utilizing more than one method in a qualitative research inquiry, but the pitfalls of relying on one methodology alone, as well. For example, if we had selected only the narrative approach without the holistic approach of examining menopause within the reproductive life course, the results of the analysis would have been misleading. In fact, many key cultural factors would not have been identified, and the study would have therefore been incomplete. Comparing similarities and differences of responses help minimize overgeneralization, provide depth to the analysis, and suggest hypotheses for further research.

Likewise, had the focus groups been the sole source of information on breast-feeding and the time and reasons for early supplementation, the realities of women's work and the cultural factors that affect breast milk production among rural farming Cameroonian women would have been overlooked.

Some Lessons Learned

The use of participant-observation in both examples presented in this chapter reveal differences between verbal responses and social action. This is an important element of an anthropological approach and is essential in both medical and non-medical fields of research. By participating in the everyday life of the women, the researcher has the opportunity to engage in general conversation with women on different topics related to being a woman, and is able to gather insights into the complexity of women's everyday lives. The ambiguous relationship between language and action fundamentally informs anthropological research using participant-observation. While qualitative health research often fails to distinguish between normative statements, narrative reconstructions, and actual practices, anthropological practice, by "situating" an interviewee's statements and the circumstances of the interview in the broader context of that person's life, helps ensure awareness of these distinctions. Participant- observation may not always be feasible or appropriate given constraints on time, funding, and expertise, but these critical methodological lessons from anthropology are transferable. First, words cannot be taken at face value; transcripts of interviews are less reliable for developing an understanding of relative importance of different attitudes or responses to a particular topic.

Second, naturally arising informal situations involving talk and action are sometimes more useful than formal interviews in highlighting the study topic.

Researchers who study human behavior must be open to all methods, avenues, and possibilities to fully understand the question(s) at hand. When studying human behavior, using both qualitative and quantitative research approaches is important to understanding the complicated dynamics of health and illness.

Summary Points

- Anthropology examines biological, cultural, ecological, linguistic, and historical factors to improve our understanding of health and illness.
- The research methods of anthropology are comparative and holistic, integrating the various aspects of health and disease.
- A key anthropological contribution to health and aging research lies in its empirically-based grasp of the context-specific nature of social processes, focusing on the complex details of everyday life.
- Anthropological practice situates an interviewee's statements and the circumstances of the interview in the broader context of that person's life, helping to ensure awareness of distinctions between normative statements, narrative reconstructions, and actual practices.

References

1) Lambert, H. and McKevitt, C. Anthropology in Health Research: From Qualitative Methods to Multidisciplinarity. *British Medical Journal.* 2002; 325: 210-213.

2) Cooper, H., Booth, K., and Gill, G. Using Combined Research Methods for Exploring Diabetes Patient Education. *Patient Education and Counseling.* 2003; 51 (1): 45-52.

3) Vidich, A.J. and Lyman, S.M. Qualitative Methods: Their History in Sociology and Anthropology. In Denzin, N.K. and Lincoln, Y.S. (Eds.). *The Landscape of Qualitative Research: Theories and Issues* (2nd Ed.). Thousand Oaks, CA: Sage Publications, 2003, pp. 55-129.

4) Brown, P.J., Barrett, R.L., and Padilla, M.B. Medical Anthropology: An Introduction to the Fields. In Brown, P.J. (Ed). *Understanding and Applying Medical Anthropology.* Mountain View, CA: Mayfield Publishing, 1998, pp. 1-10.

5) Lambert, H. Encyclopedia of Social and Cultural Anthropology. *Medical Anthropology.* London: Roultledge, 1996: 358-61.

6) Moore, L.G., Van Arsdale, P.W., Glittenberg, J.E., and Aldrich, R.B. *The Biocultural Basis of Health. Expanding Views of Medical Anthropology.* Prospect Heights, Illinois: Waveland Press, 1980, pp. 1-10.

7) Hahn, R.A. Anthropology and the Enhancement of Public Health Practice. In Hahn, R.A. (Ed). *Anthropology in Public Health: Bridging Differences in Culture and Society.* New York: Oxford University Press, 1999; pp. 3-24.

8) Trostle, J.A. and Sommerfeld, J. Medical Anthropology and Epidemiology. *Annual Review of Anthropology,* 1996; 25:253-74

9) Sokolovsky, J. (Ed.) *The Cultural Context of Aging: World-Wide Perspectives.* 2nd Edition. Greenwood: Bergin and Garvey, 1997.

10) Hurwicz, M.L. Anthropology, Aging and Health. *Medical Anthropology Quarterly.* 1995; 9 (2): 143-145.

11) Schoenberg, N. A Convergence of Health Beliefs: An 'Ethnography of Adherence' of African-American Rural Elders with Hypertension. *Human Organization.* 1997; 56 (2):174-81.

12) Helman, C.G. *Culture, Health and Illness* (3rd edition). Oxford: Butterworth-Heinmann Ltd., 1994.

13) Spradley, J.P. *The Ethnographic Interview*. New York: Holt, Rinehart, and Winston, 1979.

14) Narayan, K. and George, K.M. Personal and Folk Narrative as Cultural Representation. In Holstein, J.A. and Gubrium, J.F. (Eds). *Inside Interviewing: New Lenses, New Concerns*. Thousand Oaks, CA: Sage Publications, 2003, pp. 449-465.

15) Coffey, A. *The Ethnographic Self –Fieldwork and Representation of Identity*. London: Sage Publications, 1999

16) Spradley, J.P. *Participant Observation*. New York: Holt, Rinehart, and Winston, 1980.

17) Singer, M. The Application of Theory in Medical Anthropology: An Introduction. *Medical Anthropology Quarterly*. 1992; 14:1-8.

18) Clyde, M.J. Case and situation analysis. *Social Review*. 1983; 31:187-211.

19) Beyene, Y. *From Menarche to Menopause: Reproductive Lives of Peasant Women in Two Cultures*. Albany, NY: State University of New York, 1989.

20) Beyene, Y. and Martin, M.C. Menopausal Experiences and Bone Density of Mayan Women in Yucatan, Mexico. *American Journal of Human Biology* 2001; 13:505-511.

21) Lock, M. *Encounters with Aging: Mythologies of Menopause in Japan and North America*. Berkeley: University of California Press, 1993.

22) du Toit, B.M. *Aging and Menopause among Indian South African Women*. Albany: State University of New York, 1990.

23) Ellison, P.T. Advances in Human Reproductive Ecology. *Annual Reviews of Anthropology*. 1994; 23: 255-275

24) Ettinger, B., Genant, H.K., and Cann, C.E. Long-Term Estrogen Replacement Therapy Prevents Bone Loss and Fractures. *Annals of Internal Medicine* 1985; 102:319-324.

25) Grey, A.B., Cundy, T.F., Reid, I.R. Continuous Combined Estrogen/Progestin Therapy is Well Tolerated and Increases Bone Density at the Hip and Spine in Postmenopausal Osteoporosis. *Clinical Endocrinology*. 1994; 40:671-677.

26) Elias, S.G. et al. Caloric Restriction Reduces Age at Menopause: The Effect of the 19441945 Dutch Famine. *Menopause*. 2003: 10(5): 385-6.

27) Jelliffe, D.B. and Maddocks, J. Notes on Ecological Malnutrition in the New Guinea Highlands. *Clinical Pediatrics*. 1964; 3:305-309.

28) Del Vecchio et al. Oncology and Narrative Time. *Social Science and Medicine*. 1994; *38*(6): 855-62.

29) Gordon, D. Embodying Illness, Embodying Cancer. *Culture Medicine and Psychiatry* 1990; 14:275-97.

30) WHO/UNICEF The Innocenti Declaration: Breastfeeding in the 1990s: A Global Initiative, co-sponsored by the United States Agency for International Development (AID) and the Swedish International Development Authority (SIDA), held at the Spedale degli Innocenti. Florence, Italy, 30 July - 1 August 1990.

31) Jain, A.K. and Bongaarts, J. Breastfeeding: Patterns, Correlates, and Fertility Effects. *Study of Family Planning*. 1981; 2(3): 79-99.

32) Short, R.V., Lewis, P.R., Renfree, M.B., and Shaw, G. Contraceptive Effects of Extended Lactational Amenorrhoea: Beyond the Bellagio Consensus. *Lancet*. 1991; 337(8743): 715-7.

33) Goldman, A.S. and Garza, C. Future Research in Human Milk. *Pediatric Research*. 1987; 22(5): 493-6.

34) Beyene, Y. Workload Demands and Lactational Metabolic Load of Farming Women in NW Cameroon. Paper presented at 11th International Congress on Women's Health Issues, San Francisco, CA January 26-29, 2000.

35) IFAD (International Fund for Agricultural Development). West and Central Africa Division. *Assessment of Rural Poverty in West and Central Africa*. Rome. August, 1999.

36) Kinabo, J., Kamukama, E., and Bukuku, U. Seasonal Variation in Physical Activity Patterns, Energy Expenditure and Nutritional Status of Women in Rural Villages in Tanzania. *South African Journal of Clinical Nutrition*. 2003; 16(3): 95-101.

37) Bidinger, P.D., Nag, B., and Babu, P. Nutritional and Health Consequences of Seasonal Fluctuations in Household Food Availability. *Food and Nutrition Bulletin*. 1986; 8(1): 36-60.

38) McDade, T.W. and Worthman, C.M. The Weanling's Dilemma Reconsidered: A Biocultural Analysis of Breastfeeding Ecology. *Journal of Developmental & Behavioral Pediatrics*. 1998; 4: 286-299.

Chapter 10

State of the Art: Integrating Software with Qualitative Analysis

Raymond C. Maietta, PhD

Introduction

Integrating software with qualitative analysis presents both opportunities and challenges. This chapter draws upon my experience as President of ResearchTalk, Inc., which provides consultation on qualitative research to government, not-for-profit and academic researchers. Our main goal is to maintain the integrity of their qualitative work, a challenge that is particularly acute when researchers use qualitative software. Initially, we focus on choosing the package that best fits the needs of that particular researcher or research team. Next, we work to ease the transition to software use. This chapter focuses on integrating qualitative software into a qualitative analysis project. The two steps mentioned above are integral to the process.

There are two critical areas to consider when choosing a qualitative software package, if long-term satisfaction with that package is your goal.[*] First, the package should take advantage of the most recent computer technology. Second, the package should support a range of analytic approaches. This goal can be achieved through flexible functionality. Flexible functionality eases simple clerical tasks and supports the need to shift gears and redirect analysis when the discovery of serendipitous ideas opens new directions. The remainder of this chapter will focus on ATLAS.ti and MAXqda to demonstrate how to integrate software into research and will illuminate the strengths of these packages. Recent changes in ATLAS.ti and MAXqda clarify that the direction and decision-making of a qualitative analysis project is, and always should be, in the hands and minds of the researcher rather than the software package. Features unique to each package that allow the researcher to maintain control and review data are included below.

After reviewing software choice and defining "state of the art" for qualitative software, I provide detail of new innovations in ATLAS.ti and MAXqda. The

---

[*]Our company offers two qualitative software packages, ATLAS.ti and MAXqda, and continues to support users of ATLAS.ti, ETHNOGRAPH, HyperResearch, MAXqda and NVIVO 2.0. As new versions of ETHNOGRAPH, HyperResearch, and NVIVO are released, we will consider expansion of our product offerings. At the time of this writing (June of 2005), ATLAS.ti and MAXqda have distanced themselves from their competition in important ways for qualitative researchers.

remainder of the chapter features an analysis process I call "Sort and Sift: Think and Shift," to illustrate how qualitative software is used throughout the life of a qualitative research project.

Choosing Software and Defining "State of the Art"

Choosing Software

The five points discussed in this section will help you make informed decisions about qualitative software choice and introduction into your work.

Popularity by Marketing and Word of Mouth is NOT a Reliable Strategy.[1]

Qualitative software developers do not advertise consistently, and all operate with different marketing budgets and expertise. How your colleagues work with software may be very different than how you choose to work. For example, some users buy software to analyze data that are part of a mixed-methods project, while others use software to analyze in-depth interviews. Depending on the case, the features and functions required will vary greatly. Additionally, your colleagues may be more or less adept at the computer than you are and may be attracted to or distracted by issues in interface design differently from you. While some ATLAS.ti users love the wide range of functions available via context menus (right mouse clicks), others who do not make use of context menus find them distracting. Stylistic rather than substantive issues can result in harsh and perhaps unfair criticism of a software package. Carefully measure feedback from colleagues to prevent premature rejection of a package. Ask a colleague to introduce you to the package and appraise it for you. A detailed discussion about the software will help you gauge if others prioritize software preferences in the same way as you.

Most Packages Offer Similar Features

Do not expect major differences between qualitative software packages. Most of the major commercially available packages that support theory building offer the same core functionality, a major advantage. Each package mentioned in this chapter makes basic components of most major qualitative research methods easier via the use of software. They allow you to code textual data into the categories you create either before or during your reading of text. Each also offers easy tools for retrieval of text coded to any category within your entire project. This retrieval might be for one code at a time or for times where more than one code is applied to the same text (other Boolean and Proximity operators facilitate more complex patterns of code combinations within and across data documents). Each program also includes a comprehensive system for writing and reviewing memos and incorporating demographic variables into your analysis.

Don't Expect Software to Change Your Method

Don't look to the computer as a magic elixir. Any form of artificial intelligence or computer-aided programming depends on patterns in data and formulaic approaches applied by the computer that do not match the unpredictable nature of qualitative data. If your computer program codes for you, you miss the fine discoveries that result from your frustrations with the coding process. Often, the frustrations that characterize qualitative work are the place where we find our stories. Software should stay in the background as we direct what is done when and record what we see and think.

Consider Analysis Approach Before Software Choice

You direct the show and should impose your method on the package. Come to software with an understanding of how you need to treat your data. Think about your first steps as data become available to you. If you read text, highlight interesting passages and write notes before you code; this exercise can be done on screen. If you create codes that result from your highlighted segments and written notes, replicate that process on-screen. Alternatively, if you are testing a theory and have a set of codes that represent ideas in that theory, and then create those codes before you read text, as you find passages consistent with those ideas, code them to those categories.

Expect Qualitative Software to Take Advantage of Functionality Available in Other Software Programs

The six features discussed here position qualitative software as a practical tool that facilitates comfortable interaction with your data.

1) Interaction with other software programs—The ability to import and export ASCII text (generic computer language) marked the easiest way to transfer files between qualitative software programs and Microsoft products like WORD and Excel. The ability to export frequency tables directly to Excel has been a feature in ETHNOGRAPH for some time. HyperResearch exports data matrices to CHIP (a simple statistical program). N6 exports code lists to the modeling programs Inspiration and Decision Explorer. ATLAS.ti 5.0 exports to SPSS directly. NVIVO introduced the ability to import rich text files that preserve document formats. MAXqda and ATLAS.ti allow rich text files that contain graphics; the only size limits are those set by our computers. This feature invites interaction with a range of documents including information from websites and reports from organizations. Video, audio, and graphic files can be analyzed directly in ATLAS.ti and HyperResearch. ATLAS.ti and MAXqda are also taking advantage of XML and HTML programming language to enhance the types of reports and interactivity of reports we export from these programs. Unfortunately, MAC users find fewer options for qualitative analysis software. While HyperResearch and HyperQual can be used, they do not offer the same dynamic options as the PC-based ATLAS.ti and MAXqda. MAC users must choose programs with less flexibility or use a PC emulator with a PC-based program.

2) Use of color and visual tools—The colored pencil has been a tool that qualitative analysts have used strategically for years. Individual colors are

used consistently to represent codes or themes. This approach allows a researcher to quickly scan a coded document to see where specific codes occur in the document and where combinations of colors reveal more than one code of interest occurring at the same time. MAXqda is the first package to effectively simulate this process on-screen. Users can designate any of eleven different colors to each code. When a code is applied to text, the color stripe that appears in the margin alongside the code will be that designated color. For example, if I use the color blue for the code "friend," I will know that whenever I see that color in the margin the code friend is applied to that text.

Another new feature in MAXqda is color coding. If I apply the "magenta" code, the highlighted text is changed to that color font and the code magenta is applied. Other programs allow users to change the color of fonts, but do not allow the user to gather everything labeled with a color code. This function allows the use of these codes in a number of ways including as "temperature" measures of different ideas.

In ATLAS.ti, the "import neighbors" function brings all text segments coded to a chosen code category into a diagram. Each segment occupies its own tile. An analyst can shift the tiles to contemplate a next level of coding or text treatment. For example, in a study of life satisfaction, we had a generic code for "challenges." When we brought all segments coded into one diagram, we were able to separate financial, physical, and emotional challenges into different places in the diagram to consider each set individually and in combination.

3) Discrete control of text segments—A fair criticism of qualitative software is that it is built in a way that privileges coding as a central component of an analysis strategy. As a result, qualitative researchers become adept at diagnosing patterns across a data set at the expense of understanding the holistic meaning of a document and recognizing the power of individual statements in text. The "quotation" in ATLAS.ti provides opportunities to use text segments to address this issue. Essentially, any segment of text a researcher marks can become a computer object. This feature allows interaction with data that do not require categorization. You can begin an analysis by simply reading and marking text. MAXqda 2.0 has introduced color codes that simulate the off-screen work researchers do with a highlight pen. With these functions, both programs invite researchers to feature important text segments in their text review and reporting. Taken together, highlighted text segments help portray the overall flow and essence of a data document. They can also be reviewed as a transition to coding. More detail on interaction with these features will be discussed later.

4) Reliability—Can you trust the program to perform as expected? If you encounter a problem, can you track down the source and find resolution? No qualitative software program has an on-demand technical support service. However, all programs either have a listserve or email system built to address problems, and they score high in this regard. Nonetheless, there

is always a possibility for conflict with rapid advances and unpredictable releases of upgrades to Windows operating systems by Microsoft. We have found that developers are very responsive and quickly release patches to fix the problems.

5) Backup Facilities—It is critical to have the ability to back up an entire project in one file and save that file easily to a flash or jump drive and/or send it via email. This facility is more of a priority in qualitative software and now exists in ATLAS.ti, MAXqda, and NVIVO. It should also be possible to set up a project with ease, understand where files need to be saved for work with your data, and know where the files you save are located on your hard drive or network. MAXqda is straightforward in this regard. Other programs are more challenging.

6) Convenience Features—When qualitative software developers take full advantage of functionality available in a Windows environment, our use of the program is facilitated. When qualitative researchers work without a computer, they keep important resources at hand and in easy reach. Highlight pens or colored pencils, in a carefully chosen array of colors, are in their right place, and each is assigned its own idea to mark. Sticky notes, index cards, file folders, tape, space on walls, etc., are all available and ready to use. Qualitative software programs should be designed in similar fashion. When a researcher has an idea about what he or she has just read, noting that idea should be a seamless process. The design of a package can make this very easy. As qualitative software evolves, pragmatism should be paramount. It is important that software makes what we do easier so our insights are not lost to a search for a feature that is not well placed or easily accessible. This area is one in which ATLAS.ti and MAXqda excel.

Easy to find features and functions—Useful menus, toolbars with easy to interpret icons, and context menus make our work move along more smoothly. For example, "context menus" are found when we right click anywhere on our screen. In qualitative software, context menus should effectively lead us to common functions. A right click on a code in the margin area of ATLAS.ti reveals a range of potential places to explore while you work with your text. For example, if you code a section of text to "pivotal moments," you can right click on it in the right margin and easily write a note about your growing understanding of the code. If you are curious about how you are using the code, you can move through all other segments coded to the category. Other options are also available. The right mouse directs researchers to the "tools" they need for the next steps in both ATLAS.ti and MAXqda.

Drag and drop—In the spirit of "let me take it from here and also put it here," drag and drop allows ready movement of key ideas into memos, code categories, and/or diagrams. The availability of drag-and-drop functionality further "pushes the envelope" of the power of software as pragmatic tool.

Windows Management—Imagine if another person sat at your desk or in the room where you work with your qualitative data. Would it be a problem for you if things were moved around? The physical placement of what we review and the tools we use during that review are critical. Increasingly, the user can control the look of the computer screen and the placement of items on the screen. The foundation of the MAXqda interface is a four-window screen that is easy to adapt. Only one of the four windows needs to open at any one time, and it is easy to make adjustments to the screen according to user preference. ATLAS.ti 5.0 contains specific windows management features to make setting the screen to your preference easy and powerful. For example, "always on top" will keep a memo (or other chosen window) open even if you move to and perform functions within other windows on the screen. "Rollup mode" will keep only the title of a window open until you move your mouse to the title bar. Features like "always on top" and "rollup mode" enhance access to critical pieces of work that, when put aside temporarily, will still be at our fingertips at any point.

Defining "State of the Art"

When defined by researchers and not by computer programmers, "State of the Art" for qualitative software has less to do with sophisticated computer features than the ability for a user to maintain control and direction of an analysis using software. Built well, qualitative software facilitates sensible data organization, thorough memo writing, and dynamic access to our work that encourages us to think out loud in ways we might not otherwise do.

Two main outcomes really matter when using software. First, qualitative software should free you from administrative tasks in a manner that allows you to focus on your text and record your reactions to it. This benefit should far outweigh the predictable frustrations of integrating a new software program into a project. Second, as a result of the first point, you should enjoy the process. You do not have to find creative ways to name codes to show the relationship between code categories. You do not need to group codes into a hierarchy. When you write a memo or comment, you should be confident that you can easily retrieve it. It should be straightforward to record your reasons for changing your mind. These points are facilitated by a program that is designed to accommodate flexibility to review and mark text while retrieving, reviewing, and processing the work you do. The following discussion shows how qualitative researchers work through their projects and how ATLAS.ti and MAXqda meet the goals discussed above and set the standard for "State of the Art."

An Approach to Data Analysis—Sort and Sift: Think and Shift

Any qualitative software package can be used for almost any approach to qualitative data analysis. Further, as in research without a computer, there is no right approach for qualitative research and no step-by-step plan to follow for data analysis. A strong qualitative software program is flexible and facilitates fluid movement between reviewing the material and recording your reactions to that material in the form of highlights, categorization, and written notes. This foundation invites a wide range of qualitative options.

To demonstrate the flexibility and fluidity of ATLAS.ti and MAXqda, I use a qualitative analysis approach I call, "Sort and Sift: Think and Shift." This brief introduction to the method illustrates the benefits derived from the use of software. The Sort and Sift technique encourages frequent movement between thorough review of data with recording of ideas that emerge during review and stepping back to review and reflect on content and process used during data analysis. The approach is a process that involves two recurrent phases of a cycle of data analysis. (See Figure 1) The first phase is called "Diving In." Get into your data as quickly as possible. Read, review, recognize, and record. The second phase is called "Stepping Back." This phase encourages you to stop to review where you are. Reflect and re-strategize. Then dive back into what you have done and recognize what is new.

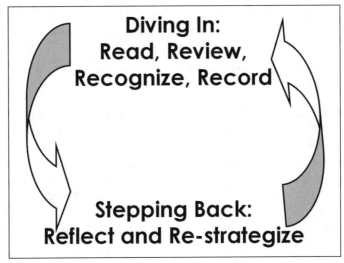

Figure 1. The Sort and Sift Cycle.

The method discourages a linear approach to qualitative data analysis. Your work, your data, and your self are all subjects of study. John Seidel,[2] the creator of ETHNOGRAPH, describes a process of "Collecting, Noticing, and Thinking" that is at the core of the Sort and Sift method. It also encourages constant movement between what we have in front of us, what we notice, and how we process both. (See Figure 2) Notice the flow of the arrows in the diagram he uses to demonstrate the qualitative analysis process in the appendix of the ETHNOGRAPH manual.

The following sections of this chapter include discussions of "Diving Into Data" and "Stepping Back." Both phases are always necessarily intertwined. A part of thorough investigation of data is to step back while in the depth of data exploration. Remember that you are considering ideas that evolve. Looking at them as you work with them facilitates how you monitor and develop ideas. This process allows you to consider how you are thinking about and relating to these developing notions as well.

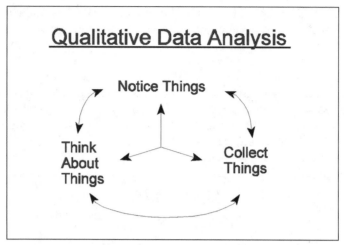

Figure 2. Seidel's "Collecting, Noticing, and Thinking."

Diving Into Data: Open Review, Memo Writing, and Codebook Evolution

"How do I get started?" is a reasonable question for people new to qualitative software. "How would you approach your data if you did not have a software program" is a reasonable response. If users are not driven by a specific method, like grounded theory, we encourage them to find an innocent point of entry into their data. In the next section, two different approaches that can be taken upon initial review of data, highlighting text and coding, are demonstrated. During each discussion, options to write memos are described as well.

Highlighting Text

MAXqda 2.0 recently introduced a new function that adds a convenient twist to the simple process of using a highlight pen and writing notes in the margin area of a document. Four different "color codes" can be applied to selected text segments and serve as an electronic highlight pen. When you highlight text and apply a color code, the font of the marked text is changed to the color of the code, and the code name then appears in the margin of the document. You can also write a memo about the segment. A memo icon will be placed in the margin to indicate that a memo is there. (See Figure 3)

Other qualitative software programs allow you to change the color of text in your documents and/or highlight selected text. MAXqda offers a further advantage beyond the ability to mark the text segment. Every segment marked with the same color code is gathered to that particular code category. You can then go back and review all text coded (highlighted) with the magenta code. As you "step back" to process your initial review of text, you can easily move through each segment you marked with a specific color to reconsider your findings and/or question why certain types of segments draw your attention. While you review, you are returned to the original text to see your original memos and review those as well.

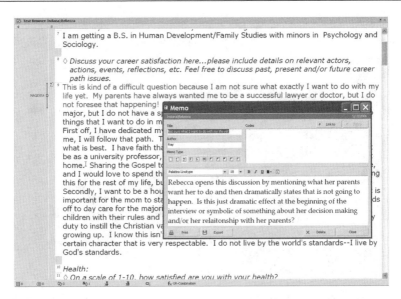

Figure 3. MAXqda 'magenta' color code and memo with question mark icon for a memo.

The "quotation" in ATLAS.ti also serves as an electronic highlight pen and offers other interesting options. Before you code, you can highlight text and make it a quotation. This process is equivalent to highlighting text off-screen. A bracket is placed in the margin area of the document indicating the beginning and end points of the quotation. Each quotation can be named, and you can write a comment about each one. All quotations are placed in an easily accessible list. As you examine the list, you start to see the story of the data document under review and may begin to think about codes suggested from this reading.

The quotation manager, which I prefer to place on the right side of my screen, shows a list of every quotation I created while reading a journal interview "George" typed as part of a study of life satisfaction. (See Figure 4) I can read the list of quotes to consider a potential code list and to get a profile of what I learned about George through the interview. As I review each quotation, I can call up the comments I wrote about them. From this list of quotations, I see that relationships are central to George's life as he makes statements that are both general about relationships and specific about friends, family, and romantic partners. He discusses future interests about wanting to be a movie director. Our final code list includes specific codes for different key actors and a general category for "interests." These codes emerged from our first read of George's document.

ATLAS.ti offers other "stepping back" tools in addition to reviewing code names for a document profile and potential codes. This program also features network diagrams to explore and represent relationships between and among documents, quotes, codes, memos, and other objects in ATLAS.ti. The diagram below shows a network view for George's interview. (See Figure 5) As we read George's document, we noted that his discussion was compartmentalized into two areas: relationships and a desire to be a movie director. Each tile in the

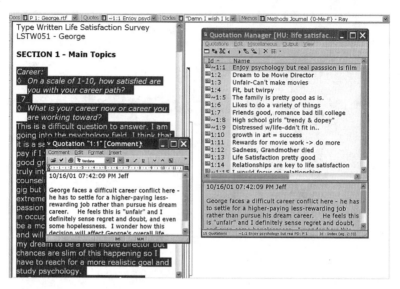

Figure 4. ATLAS.ti Quotation Manager, highlighted quote, and quote comment.

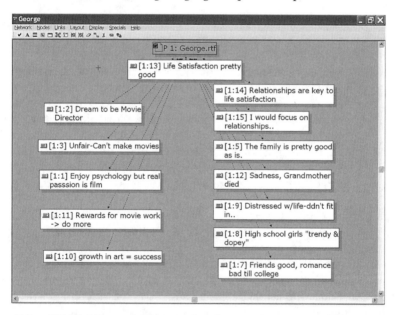

Figure 5. An ATLAS.ti Network Diagram that shows a document and important quotes marked, named and arranged to convey the document profile.

diagram is a quotation to which we gave a unique name. Unlike the process for coding, here we wanted to create a short name to summarize the quote and capture the essence of the statement rather than note patterns and group quotes.

We design "Episode Profiles" about George by arranging the tiles in a network diagram in an order that portrays the "shape" of his discussion. We also write a comment about each diagram as part of this profile to represent what we learn about each person in our study. Episode profiles provide powerful points for discussion and serve as comparative tools as we think about differences across our population. This level of analysis generates valuable information. What you learn and show about each case is as important as what you learn and show about your code categories. Specific, detailed quote names help capture the dynamic nature of each statement featured in the diagram. The flexibility of the network diagram allows us to play with what we are learning. While George's diagram is in columns, we represented the story told by a woman in our study by moving her tiles into a circle. A third woman had one quote from which several other key quotes emerged. Her diagram simulated a shooting star.

Color codes are unique to MAXqda. Discrete use of quotations as objects that can be named, commented on, and included in network diagrams as described here is unique to ATLAS.ti.

Memo Writing

Memo writing is probably the most common qualitative task we avoid when we feel time pressure. It is also the best way to develop a deep relationship to your work. Memos facilitate out loud thinking. Memos should be treated as living, breathing documents where ideas evolve. We should write something about every aspect of our projects. This writing does not have to be elegant or brilliant, but should capture your thoughts. Memos should be reviewed and revised frequently to monitor emerging ideas.

When we work off-screen, we develop methods for putting memos about different items in their proper places. We may attach a piece of paper to each file folder that contains an interview, focus group, or field note to keep reflections, summaries, and questions regarding each document. If we use file folders for code categories, we may write notes on the folder or on attached pages. We use the margins to write comments on text. Separate tablets may be assigned to major project memos like methods notes, ToDo lists, and/or emerging questions.

Qualitative software is built to simulate this notation process. ATLAS.ti comments and MAXqda memos can be written for each quotation and/or code we use to simulate notes in the margin of a document. These items are like industrial strength sticky notes that stay with that text wherever you reference it. If you code a segment to the codes for "health" and "pivotal moments," you will see an icon to access your note while you review the segments coded to either code category. As is the case in most of the major packages on the market, you can also write comments or memos (the terms vary in the different packages) that attach to a document, code category, or other major item in your project. You can also simulate having a tablet for major project memos by writing memos for the project that are available via memo system managers in ATLAS.ti and MAXqda. Since the memos and comments you write are accessible and editable, return to review and change them, and consider the meaning of each change in a methods journal.

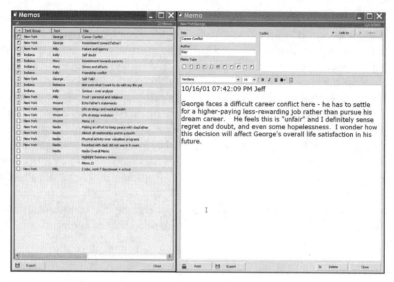

Figure 6. The MAXqda memo manager and a MAXqda memo.

Throughout the sections on highlighting text and codework you see references to how to access memos and comments. They should be readily available. You access them the same way you construct them, to review, add to and adjust.

ATLAS.ti and MAXqda also contain special access tools for you to step back and review memos. This window shows (See Figure 6) the MAXqda memo manager and a MAXqda memo. The memo manager lists every memo in the project and is sortable. When you write a memo, you can classify it by type. For example, you can use an icon with a "T" on it to indicate a memo that contains a theoretical notion. You can then sort your memo list to move to those memos. ATLAS.ti also has a memo manager. In ATLAS.ti, notes about specific objects in the project like codes, documents, and quotes are called comments. While comments are not accessible via the memo manager, you can use filtering to see the objects that contain comments. Each item with a comment is also indicated with a marker (a tilde [~] in a list or a colored triangle on a quotation marker in the document margin area).

Codework

One debate in the field of qualitative analysis is whether coding is analysis. When done right, it absolutely is. Analysis proceeds during the coding phase. Qualitative analysis requires multiple passes through each data piece. During each phase we should keep our "memo mind" active. Let thoughts develop. Record and refine them. Think of writing as a comfortable companion to coding. Carefully learn the layout of a software program to understand where necessary tools are located. When you code to a category and realize that the coded segment is a cornerstone example of that idea, copy it directly to a memo. Similarly, when you code to a category and think that a section of text may or may not fit a code category, write a note and explore other places that have been coded to that category to understand how segments may or may not fit together. This section details two key aspects of the design of ATLAS.ti and MAXqda that facilitate active codework: 1) a screen view that encourages flexible, fluid movement between text (and/or videos, graphics, audio), codes, memos, etc.; and 2) An active code book that offers flexible ways to view and question category status.

Codework Screen View

Both ATLAS.ti and MAXqda offer flexible options for how to set up your screen while you work. Much as individual qualitative researchers make decisions about how to set up their desk and office space, the options available for screen setup accommodate different work processes. Each program shares important design elements. The following illustration from ATLAS.ti demonstrates how tools are utilized to work through a data piece conveniently. (See Figure 7)

The margin area directly next to the body of the data piece under review displays codes and markers where applications begin and end. The margin area in both ATLAS.ti and MAXqda is active. Right clicking on any item exposes a context menu that lists a choice of functions for coding and document review.

In the ATLAS.ti screenshot pictured here, the option, "list quotations" is highlighted within the margin area context menu. In this case, the highlighted text is coded to the category "challenges." When we analyzed the category, we battled with what it meant and how to use it. The list quotations function gave

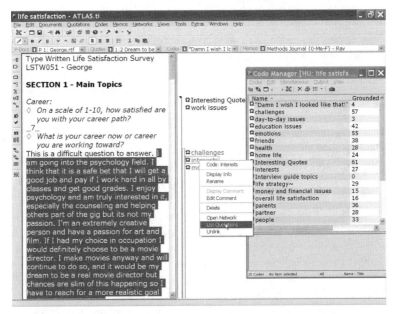

Figure 7. Personalized Workspace - one possible setup for the ATLAS.ti screen.

us access to every instance we coded as "challenges." By scanning these instances to assess the idea "challenges," we considered what we learned from it. As we reviewed instances, we could also access a comment function to write notes about what we learned, and a rename function to refine the name of the code.

Reading and reviewing data inspires unanticipated reactions and reflections. Some reactions are related to the immediate data while others concern items we have wrestled with previously. Qualitative software programs offer a comprehensive toolkit of resources needed to review a data piece. Only ATLAS.ti and MAXqda include the complete set of items listed here:

- Easy to read code names in the margin area.
- Clear markers indicating the beginning and ending of each code application. MAXqda only—these markers are color coded in colors determined by the user. Each time a code or group of codes appears in the document margin, the stripe for that code becomes the color you set in the code system window. MAXqda is the only program that controls colors of code markers by code category and lets the user determine the color for each code.
- An active margin area providing ready access to a range of functions to perform during document review.
- The ability to open important windows to accompany document review (code lists, document lists, lists of key text segments) via a right mouse click or click of an icon.
- Convenient drag-and-drop functionality to link key items within your project.
- Straightforward functionality to do and undo tasks.
- Document editing.
- Memo access via clear icons and mouse clicks.
- On-screen review that occurs in the same screen view as original work with a data document.
- Ready access to all segments coded to a category while coding a particular data document.

While this list is not exhaustive, it represents a spectrum of activity that may occur while coding. The availability of this flexible set of tools increases the likelihood that your ideas are not lost.

Active Code Book

Code books evolve. Therefore, it is necessary to have an easy to access code book and the ability both to change codes in or out of the code book (change codes from the document margin area as described in the previous section) and to see your code list in different ways. The picture here shows two different views of a code list in MAXqda. (See Figure 8)

The list on the left shows codes that we have organized into categories and subcategories. To the right of each code is a number indicating a count of text

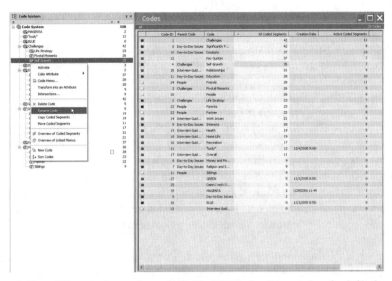

Figure 8. Two different views of a code list in MAXqda. View 1 (on the left) shows the standard code system view. View 2 (on the right) shows a frequency of codes list sorted by frequency for only active text segments.

segments coded to each category. This feature is available in both ATLAS.ti and MAXqda, but not in all programs discussed here. In addition, each code name is preceded by an icon that displays the color you choose to associate with that code in the document margin area. Categories and subcategories can be arranged and rearranged via drag-and-drop. When the code list is open alongside a data document, coding by drag-and-drop is easy.

Both ATLAS.ti and MAXqda allow you to view and code from a code list view that is organized by category and subcategory. In ATLAS.ti you can opt to code by list as well. In MAXqda and ATLAS.ti, codes can also be listed in a view that can be sorted by code name and/or by a range of other code characteristics. This flexibility inspires different ways to think about your code list and how it is used. You can sort code lists by authors assigned to each code or by frequency of application. The code view on the right side of the screenshot here is sorted by frequency for documents of New Yorkers. Flexible sorting and filtering, available in most qualitative software packages, allows you to critically compare: "Are my coding patterns for documents from New Yorkers different than my coding patterns for documents for people from Indiana?"

The ability to think out loud about code categories helps your growing understanding of your project. Changing how we view and ask questions about our code list assists this process. For example, looking at your code list in a sortable list or organized into categories and subcategories inspires important questions about the content and direction of your analysis. When you decide to make changes to code names, code definitions, how codes are grouped, new codes or codes to delete, these changes can be made easily from within the code managers. (Please see the context menu in the MAXqda screenshot in this section.)

- *Working with demographics*—all qualitative software packages offer the ability to categorize data documents at the demographic level. For example, you can indicate which documents belong to sub-categories of gender, job tenure, income and state of residence and examine those documents by one or more of these categories to assess the effect of demographic variables on various situations in your data.
- *Special feature*—Weighting codes as a heuristic device in MAXqda—You can modify the weight of each coded instance in MAXqda. Weight scores vary from 1–100. You set the default weight for segments that are not explicitly weighted. In the following example, we apply a weight score to a text segment coded to the category "interests." (See Figure 9) Our default weight is set at one. In this case we used code weighting to signify indications of preference in a series of text segments. We wanted to isolate those from other instances coded to this category.

For each of the stronger instances, we changed the weight to a number from 75–100. This change allowed us to organize our report of all items coded to interests by weight score. While our goal was not to declare the meaning and implications of different weighted discussions of interests, we were able to look at the higher weights to see what we learned from text where the participant made explicit efforts to declare the importance of an area of interest. For example, in reviewing the statement, "My life would be incomplete without music," the weighted segments revealed that concrete indications of importance happened more often during discussions of recreation and activities shared with key actors in the participant's life. The nature of these discussions was also consistent with a general theme in our study of life satisfaction that while people don't discuss life satisfaction per se, they describe their strategies for getting through the day.

Stepping Back: Review and Representation

Throughout the section on "Diving In" to data, references to stepping back to enhance the process of data review were made. This "talk back" between

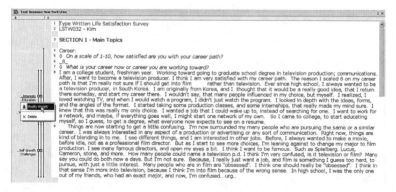

Figure 9. Code weights can be modified in MAXqda by right clicking on a code stripe in the code margin area.

what we review for the first time and our developing ideas of what has gone before is critical. In addition, there are times when we need to stop to consider preliminary thoughts about the project overall. I strongly advise that you use the tools outlined here after reviewing three to five documents rather than waiting until you have reviewed every document in your data set. Review them again after significant chunks of work are done. In this way, you allow your thoughts to move back and forth between the discrete and the whole.

Four "Stepping Back" exercises are discussed here: code review, both in output reports and on-screen, filtering by demographics, exploring combinations of codes, and diagramming ideas

Code review

Don't expect reports generated from a qualitative software program to be conclusive. In ATLAS.ti, they are aptly called "outputs." You can output the text of a document, or as pictured here, every quotation (text segment) coded to a code category. (See Figure 10) The report below is for the code "education." Note that the first instance of the output is shown in the window and begins with the text P1:George.rtf. This text indicates that this coded instance comes from George's interview. Below this main information line is a code line. This line indicates all code categories where this segment is coded. Take advantage of all information in an output report. In this case, think about the co-occurrence of categories. Perhaps you will find something new and unexpected or information that confirms an idea you are exploring. The text segment is

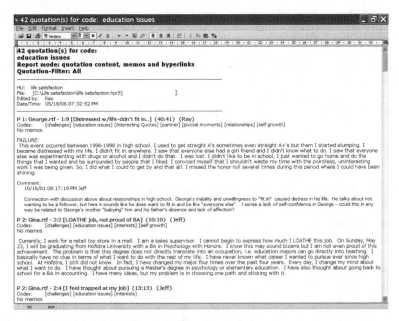

Figure 10. An ATLAS.ti Code Output Report that includes a comment written to one of the quotations coded to the selected code.

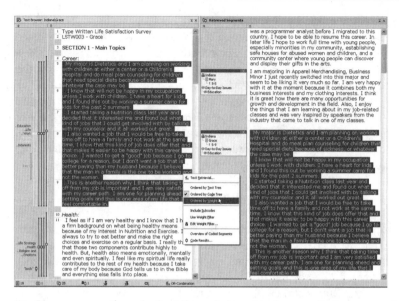

Figure 11. Users can specify and adjust the ordering of text segments that appear in the MAXqda 'retrieved segments' window.

followed by the comment we wrote about this quotation. The output report provides a thorough account of what we did while we coded this text to "education." Use this information to inform ideas and direction of new questions.

Most information in a qualitative software program can be seen on paper or on-screen. MAXqda is particularly flexible with on-screen reports. (See Figure 11) Notice that the context menu in the window in this section provides different options for the order of items in the retrieved segments window. You can choose to review the text segments of more than one code at a time and order them by document (order by text tree), by code category (order by code), or by weight. This simple feature is a powerful and frequently more effective tool for accessing information than some more sophisticated tools featured in qualitative software programs.

Filtering by Demographics

Another simple and powerful tool in qualitative software is called filtering. If we can isolate information by major categories, draw conclusions, and then do comparisons, we can move toward understanding how different characteristics contribute to different information. For example, if gender is an important variable in our analysis, we can first indicate within our software program the appropriate gender for text from each case in our study. Then we can filter to select only text for women. Every code we read and code combination we pursue will be for women only. We can then do the same for men. The similarities and differences of these explorations will yield the content of our gender comparison.

Combinations of Codes

It is easy to assume themes exist in places where more than one code is applied to the same section of text. This assumption is more likely with qualitative software because of code combination tools built from Boolean and Proximity operators. For example, we thought that people who completed our life satisfaction interviews were "becoming their parents." To explore this notion, we used a code combination tool to find instances when we coded to both the parents' code and the self-growth code. However, the only instance of this code combination was from a woman who related going to yoga classes with her mom. We then decided to step back to ask the question in a simpler way. Dropping the assumption that we could learn about people becoming their parents only where we coded these two main categories to the same text, we retrieved both the self-growth and parents' codes and ordered the retrieved segments window by text tree. This selection allowed us to read, by data document, each segment coded to parents or self-growth in the order they appeared in the data document.

The first document we read perfectly characterized our expectation. A young woman related that when she lived at home, she couldn't wait to go to college to escape her father who she described as a military drill sergeant. Everything had to be done on time and kept in an orderly manner. This segment was coded to parents. In a later section of the document we coded to self-growth, she wrote how proud she was to listen to a speech announcing that she won an award for being a dorm leader. She described how the speech characterized her as good at keeping order and making sure things happen on time. When we then read segments coded to our categories of interest in sequence, we could see how the nature of the text about the two categories was similar. The participant didn't acknowledge the similarity as would be required if the same text was about both ideas. Instead, she gave us information about each component part of this theme, and we put the pieces together by organizing the information we were reading in a new way.

In *Computer Programs for Qualitative Data Analysis,* Weitzman and Miles[3] discuss search tools available in packages they classify as "theory building packages." Searching for combinations of codes is described as a powerful feature of these programs. Tools like the Query Tool of ATLAS.ti, the Search Procedures in ETHNOGRAPH, the Logic Machine in MAXqda, and the Search Tool in NVIVO 2.0 quickly locate all instances where more than one code was applied to the same text or in the same document in a pattern designated by the user. You can find every time Code A comes before Code B or Code A is inside Code B, when they are coded to the same text or coded in overlapping ways and more. These powerful tools are a strong argument for qualitative software. Tasks like these searches would be difficult, and in some cases impossible, to replicate off-screen.

While powerful, these tools nonetheless assume that the researcher knows what code combinations to put into a search before he or she performs it. While we may know many combinations for any project, surprise combinations are equally common.

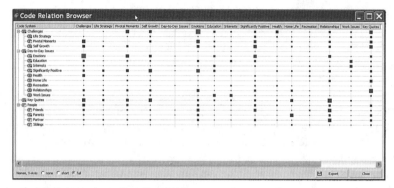

Figure 12. The MAXqda Code Relations browser showing the frequency of text segments for the selected pair of co-occurring codes.

Tools in MAXqda, ATLAS.ti, and NVIVO 2.0 let researchers see a matrix of code combinations that provide access to the associated text. The code relations browser from MAXqda is pictured here. (See Figure 12) Codes in the project (an entire code list or selection of codes designated by the user) are displayed in both columns and rows of a table. Boxes of different color and size indicate the popularity of different combinations of codes. Large red boxes indicate the most popular combinations and small blue boxes indicate less popular combinations. Double clicking on a particular box brings all instances that fit that combination to the retrieved segments window of MAXqda. The combination of education and work is highlighted in the lower right of the window below.

The motivation behind tools like the code relations browser is to provide direct access to anticipated and unanticipated code combinations in your project. It is also possible to see a list, or in some programs, like MAXqda, a matrix diagram, of all codes applied within the body of data documents. These lists facilitate the building of episode profiles described earlier in this chapter.

Diagramming Ideas

As ideas and connections between elements of our projects become more complex, keeping track of these connections becomes increasingly challenging. Qualitative researchers describe how they lay sections of field notes, interviews, and focus groups on an empty floor, wall, or table. They move index cards and cut-up sections of documents to bring complementary ideas together, and they arrange contrasting statements next to each other to vividly see contrasts. Several qualitative software programs contain facilities that qualitative researchers use to model connections between codes and documents and memos. ATLAS.ti is the only program that invites the physical movement of text segments to imitate processes described here.

The diagram in this section shows how we portray a connection between three codes, emotions, friends, and self-growth, in our life satisfaction study. While there was little explicit discussion of our main topic, these three codes comprised what we called the "life satisfaction triangle." Each code served as a

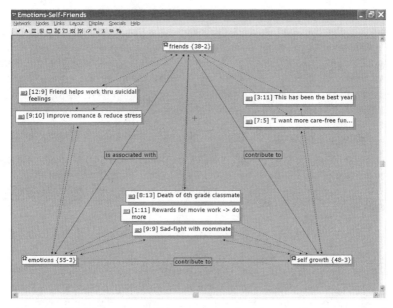

Figure 13. This ATLAS.ti network diagram shows 3 codes associated as a triangle with quotes that demonstrate the relationships between these codes.

barometer for how satisfied people were with their lives. If friendships were in disrepair, their life satisfaction seemed low. The same was true for their emotional states and how they felt about themselves. Additionally, if they focused on any of these categories, for example, engaged in self-growth activities, their life satisfaction seemed to increase.

The diagram above we constructed displays the internal associations and contributions we identified between these codes. (See Figure 13) Because ATLAS.ti treats designated text segments as computer objects, we can bring discrete text segments (quotations), to which we can apply specific names for illustrative purposes, into diagrams with codes. Including quote names helps maintain the language of our participants and adds a powerful dimension to our diagram.

Not only is this diagramming tool a representation tool, it is also an exploration tool or playground, if you will. You can bring any combination of your project's codes, quotes, memos, or documents into any diagram. Try these two powerful exercises:

Code Exploration

After you code at least ten quotations to a code category, bring that code into a network diagram. Use the import neighbors function to see the quotes you have coded to that category. Each quotation is on its own tile. Slide the tiles around to explore what you are learning about the code. When we have trouble defining and applying codes in our project, we move quotes into three columns. Column one contains quotations that exactly fit the codes to this category. Column two contains approximate "hits," and column three has quotations that do not fit. Each column teaches us about our coding patterns and helps us refine our ideas. In similar fashion, we can move the quotes coded to a broad category to sections that represent subcategories of the major code. For example, we can take quotes coded to emotions and move them to sections of the diagram we designate for each subcategory, such as happiness, guilt, and pride. After we define groupings we can code to the subcategories as well.

Shaping Episode Profiles

This same logic can be used with documents. You can import quotations that you create within a data document and can name those quotations. They can be moved to show the flow and shape of the discussion that carries through the document.

Conclusion

Be modest when you start using qualitative software. The goal of this chapter has been to allow you to picture yourself using software and guide you to choose and implement this tool in your work. Qualitative researchers who are not yet using software should think seriously about doing so. Since ATLAS.ti and MAXqda give us discrete control of the smallest units of text via the quotation, color codes, and on the spot memoing, we can invoke a range of methodological strategies in our approach to working with data in a program. Work from the core of different levels of categorization and memo writing, and value individual text segments to the same degree as any category or memo. Access stories that live inside individual data collection episodes and ride across key elements of a data set and in the process push and question your analysis approach.

Qualitative software was built to support existing approaches to data analysis. It is a pragmatic tool. While qualitative software is commonly referred to as CAQDAS (computer assisted qualitative data analysis software), I prefer the term, "qualitative software" because I object to the term, "computer assisted," leading the expression. Qualitative analysis is the most important aspect of what we do, and we do not need the computer to assist that part of it.

Ideally, the researcher should be freed by qualitative software to focus on the substance of her or his work and reactions to it. This scenario becomes more likely if we use software as an electronic organizer and dynamic access tool. The software does not give us new or different information, and the program does not do the analysis or interpretation. We remain the analysts. This bias does not preclude software enhancing methodology. When I have a reliable, dynamic organization and access tool providing visual playgrounds that encourage me to think out loud, I can think more creatively and responsibly. We are now freed from tasks that distance us from the immediacy of intimate and intellectual reaction to our work.

We don't need software to inspire dramatic findings; our participants, our data, our minds, and our audience will always be responsible for that. It can be argued that qualitative analysis can proceed from here with no further innovation to software. However, I am curious to see where we can go from here and know that there will be innovations beyond what we can currently conceptualize. We need to proceed with caution and keep pragmatic goals paramount. Create ways for the computer to reliably deal with patterned tasks that don't affect the substance of what we do. In so doing, open our options for serendipitous discovery. If software helps us be true to this task, then it is truly "state of the art."

Summary Points
- Functionality eases simple clerical tasks and supports the need to shift gears and redirect analysis when the discovery of serendipitous ideas opens new directions.
- Software should stay in the background as we direct what is done when and record what we see and think.
- The Sort and Sift technique encourages frequent movement between thorough review of data with recording of ideas that emerge during review, and stepping back to review and reflect on content and process used during data analysis.
- Software can best be used as an electronic organizer and reliable, dynamic access tool that encourages the researcher to think more creatively and responsibly.

References

1) Creswell, J.W. and Maietta, R.C. Qualitative Research. In *Handbook of Research Design and Social Measurement, 6th Edition*, Miller and Salkind, Thousand Oaks, CA. Sage, 2001.

2) Seidel, J. Appendix E: Qualitative Data Analysis. In *The ETHNOGRAPH 5.0 Manual*. Thousand Oaks, CA. Sage:1998

3) Weitzman, E. and Miles, M. *Computer Programs for Qualitative Data Analysis*. Thousand Oaks, CA. Sage, 1995.

Chapter 11

Writing a Credible and Fundable Proposal for Qualitative Research

Toni Tripp-Reimer, PhD, RN, FAAN, Stacie Salsbury Lyons, MSN RN, Nancy Goldsmith, BA, and Katherine Bussinger, BA

Introduction

Despite a substantial record of federal funding for qualitative research on aging-related topics, investigators often characterize the National Institutes of Health (NIH) as not supportive of applications employing these methods. Increasingly, qualitative health research has encountered unprecedented federal interest and encouragement in the past five years, triggered in part by several factors, including escalating health care costs, widening health disparities, unexplained practice variation, increased complexity of clinical decision-making, recognition that practice changes are not driven solely by scientific knowledge, as well as the primacy of the consumer voice.[1-5] Investigators and funding agencies have noted the limitations that traditional research approaches pose for challenging Eurocentric models of health and health behaviors. [6,7] In contrast, qualitative and community-based participatory methods that highlight the human dimension in health care by foregrounding the perceptions, experiences, and behaviors of both consumers and providers are particularly useful for addressing health care quality and system change issues. As Pope and colleagues[4] write, "Qualitative research offers a variety of methods for identifying what really matters to patients and [providers], detecting obstacles to changing performance, and explaining why improvement does or does not occur" (p. 148).

The negative characterization of the NIH toward applications using qualitative methods may be due, in part, to the overall highly competitive nature of NIH funding, as well as the highly specified format for grant applications. Unsuccessful applications may stem from confusion about the grant writing process as it pertains to proposals submitted to the NIH. In this chapter, we first outline the administrative structure, history of qualitative grant funding, and grant mechanisms of the NIH. Next, we review the grant application process and offer suggestions for completing a PHS 398 application with a qualitative focus. Finally, we comment on the NIH peer review process focusing on its five evaluation criteria of significance, approach, innovation, investigator, and environment.

National Institutes of Health

Health and social science research has seen dramatic changes over the past 40 years. The National Science Foundation (NSF) was an early leader in the funding of qualitative research, particularly in anthropology, and to a lesser degree in sociology and psychology.[5] Although few publications were initially available to guide applicants through the process of obtaining research funding for their studies,[8,9] this situation has changed considerably over the past 15 years.[10-16] Correspondingly, since the early 1990s, federal agencies and national foundations have demonstrated a growing commitment to facilitating qualitative research through a variety of mechanisms such as conferences, workshops, and monographs. The NIH, NSF, and the Agency for Health Research and Quality (AHRQ) have promoted qualitative approaches through a series of developmental initiatives and have produced visionary statements on how person-centered styles of inquiry can revolutionize our understanding and experience of wellness, illness, and health care.[17-26]

This considerable growth in federal attention to and funding for naturalistic inquiry is best understood in the context of recent innovations in health sciences and health services research, as well as an overarching concern with improving the quality of health care.[27,28] A presidential initiative to eliminate health disparities also focused attention on the ever-widening gap in markers of health status between Euro-Americans and persons of diverse ethnic/minority backgrounds.[29] Under this initiative, all federal units located within the Department of Health and Human Services (DHHS) were charged to develop and implement strategic plans to contribute to the elimination of health disparities.

While many federal agencies and private foundations (such as The John A. Hartford Foundation, Robert Wood Johnson Foundation, and The Commonwealth Foundation) finance qualitative studies conducted with older adult populations, the DHHS remains the single largest funding source for gerontological research, channeling most of its research grants through the NIH. The DHHS comprises multiple funding agencies (See Figure 1—DHHS Organizational Chart). NIH currently encompasses 27 Institutes and Centers, 24 of which have extramural grant programs (See Table 1—Institutes and Centers at the NIH). Aging-related social science research is funded by a number of these NIH entities, including National Institute on Aging (NIA), National Institute for Nursing Research (NINR), National Institute of Mental Health (NIMH), National Cancer Institute (NCI), and the National Heart, Lung, and Blood Institute (NHLBI). An extensive orientation to NIH agencies, their missions and priority areas, and funding guidelines is located on the NIH homepage at http://Grants1.nih.gov/grants.

Qualitative Research at NIH

Though talented qualitative investigators may be discouraged from submitting proposals because of critical statements such as, "NIH rarely

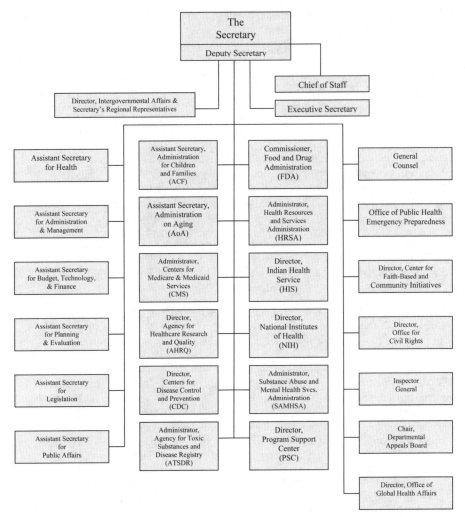

Figure 1. Department of Health and Human Services (DHHS) Organizational Chart

funds qualitative research"[30] (p. 360), NIH Institutes have funded, in fact, an array of qualitative approaches including ethnography, grounded theory, phenomenology, ethology, oral/life histories, critical and historical approaches to inquiry, as well as studies using specific qualitative techniques, including focus groups, critical incident, case study, and ethnoscience. For example, the classic "Discovery of Grounded Theory"[31] and four other books by Glaser and Strauss were made possible by a grant from the PHS, Division of Nursing (NU 00047).

Although many NIH Institutes and Centers finance investigative projects using naturalistic methods, two Institutes with particular emphasis on older adult populations are highlighted. The NIA and the NINR have taken leadership roles on varied topics in aging research, such as end-of-life,

Table 1: Institutes and Centers at the National Institutes of Health
*Extramural grant programs available

*National Cancer Institute (NCI)	*National Eye Institute (NEI)	*National Heart, Lung, and Blood Institute (NHLBI)
*National Human Genome Research Institute (NHGRI)	*National Institute on Aging (NIA)	*National Institute on Alcohol Abuse and Alcoholism (NIAAA)
*National Institute of Allergy and Infection Diseases (NIAID)	*National Institute of Arthritis and Musculoskeletal and Skin Diseases (NIAMS)	*National Institute of Biomedical Imaging and Bioengineering (NIBIB)
*National Institute of Child Health and Human Development (NICHD)	*National Institute of Deafness and Other Communication Disorders (NIDCD)	*National Institute of Dental and Craniofacial Research (NIDCR)
*National Institute of Diabetes and Digestive and Kidney Diseases (NIDDK)	*National Institute on Drug Abuse (NIDA)	*National Institute of Environmental Health Sciences (NIEHS)
*National Institute of General Medical Sciences (NIGMS)	*National Institute of Mental Health (NIMH)	*National Institute of Neurological Disorders and Stroke (NINDS)
*National Institute for Nursing Research (NINR)	*National Library of Medicine (NLM)	Center for Information Technology (CIT)
Center for Scientific Review (CSR)	*John E. Fogarty International Center (FIC)	*National Center for Complementary and Alternative Medicine (NCCAM)
*National Center on Minority Health and Health Disparities (NCMHD)	*National Center for Research Resources (NCRR)	NIH Clinical Center (CC)

informal caregiving of chronic illnesses, racial and ethnic minorities, pain management, and ethical issues, among others. A brief overview of these Institutes follows.

National Institute on Aging (NIA)

NIA was established in 1974 with a congressional mandate to coordinate the "conduct and support of biomedical, social, and behavioral research, training, health information dissemination, and other programs with respect to the aging process and diseases and other special problems and needs of the aged."[25] The NIA Strategic Goals for 2000-2005 seek to: 1) improve the health and quality of life of older people; 2) understand healthy aging processes; 3) reduce health disparities among older persons and populations; and 4) enhance resources to support high quality research. The NIA funds four areas for extramural research programs including: 1) Biology of Aging; 2) Behavioral and Social Research; 3) Neuroscience and Neuropsychology; and 4) Geriatrics and Clinical Gerontology. Within the NIA, the Behavioral and Social Research (BSR) program targets several areas of emphasis ripe for qualitatively focused initiatives: 1) health disparities; 2) aging minds; 3) increasing health expectancy; 4) health, work, and retirement; 5) interventions and behavior change; 6) genetics, behavior, and the social environment; and 7) the burden of illness and efficiency of health systems. The BSR awards the greatest ratio of research monies to investigators using naturalistic methods. Additional information about the scientific priorities of the NIA is available at the Institute's web site http://www.nia.nih.gov/.

National Institute for Nursing Research (NINR)

NINR, initially designated a NIH center in 1986, "supports clinical and basic research to establish a scientific basis for the care of individuals across the life span—from the management of patients during illness and recovery to the reduction of risks for disease and disability; the promotion of healthy lifestyles; the promotion of quality of life in those with chronic illness; and the care for individuals at the end of life."[26] This research may include elders within a family or a community context and also focuses on health disparities and the special needs of at-risk and underserved populations. NINR's funding portfolio encompasses seven areas of science, six of which are relevant for aging-related social and behavioral research using qualitative methods: 1) chronic illness and long-term care; 2) health promotion and risk reduction in adults; 3) cardiopulmonary health and critical care; 4) neurofunction and sensory conditions; 5) immune responses and oncology; and 6) end-of-life and environmental contexts. For more information about NINR priority areas go to the Institute's website at: http://ninr.nih.gov/ninr/.

Targeting an NIH Institute for a Grant Proposal

Career scientists typically develop programs of research that are funded by just one or two NIH Institutes or Centers, corresponding to the focused missions of these Institutes. Prospective applicants should know as much as possible about an Institute's characteristics in order to match a proposal with the most suitable Institute and to avoid submitting inappropriate applications. Information about an Institute's mission, interests, and goals can be culled from their strategic plans and areas of program emphasis (See Table 2—NIH Institutional Profile Characteristics).

NIH program officers strive to achieve the strongest scientific portfolio for their home Institute and are excellent resources for investigators in all

Table 2. NIH Institutional Profile Characteristics

What We Need to Know	Where to Find It
Priorities	Institute's home page website and Council reports
Grant Mechanisms	Institutes list of extramural program mechanisms
Prior History of Funding	CRISP Database
Success Rate – Payline	Annual Report
Eligibility Criteria	PA/RFP default PHS 398
$$$ Available	Federal and NIH Institutes and Centers allocations

stages of their research careers. Program officers can help interpret the nuances of calls for proposals and empower grant seekers to tailor proposals in ways that promote reviewers' receptivity and responsiveness. Before writing or submitting a proposal, applicants should consider contacting a program officer at the relevant NIH Institute or Center to: 1) determine the fit of a topic within that Institute; 2) learn about programmatic areas of interest; 3) discuss responding to a priority area of research; 4) identify funding mechanisms best suited to an investigator's project and stage of career development; and 5) discuss a proposal's potential for assignment to that Institute. Program officers may also provide feedback on ideas, abstracts, and concept papers if given sufficient time.

The Computer Retrieval of Information on Scientific Projects (CRISP) database is also an exceptional resource for learning about funding patterns and trends at NIH. CRISP is an online, searchable database of federally (DHHS) funded biomedical research projects maintained by the Office of Extramural Research and located at http://crisp.cit.nih.gov/. Using CRISP keywords, an investigator can learn about an Institute's prior history of funding particular topic areas and research methods, types and proportions of grant mechanisms used, and length of funding. The CRISP entry also indicates the name of the Initial Review Group (IRG) and information on Principal Investigators (PI) including name, state, and home institution. The two most useful features of the CRISP database are the grant abstract and the grant identification number. Activity codes, organizational codes, and definitions (2004) for extramural programs are located at: http://grants1.nih.gov/grants/funding/ac.pd.

How Often is Qualitative Research Funded by NIH?

To assess the widely held belief that qualitative research is not fundable through DHHS, we conducted an analysis of qualitative research funding at NIH and AHRQ using the CRISP database for years 1971–2005. We ran keyword searches for a variety of terms associated with qualitative methods and data collection techniques; removed false positives resulting from the use of homographs, such as "phenomenological," particularly as it characterizes mental illness, and "qualitative," particularly as it characterizes imaging, gene sequencing, and laboratory cultures; and we sorted the output by type and mechanism. Our review indicated that four NIH Institutes and the AHRQ alone funded over 1,000 new qualitative research grants in this time period. Of these grants, over one-third was funded in only the past 5 years; further about one-third of the grants were entirely qualitative with two-thirds mixed method. These grants were nearly evenly divided between Research (R) and Training/Development (F & K) categories (these are discussed below). The Institutes varied by type of grant awarded with NIA primarily funding research grants (R01 & R03), NIMH funding both research (R01 & R03) and training (F31 & K), and NINR also funding research (R01 & R15) and training (F31) awards.

Table 3 depicts the number of new grants with abstracts containing the methodological and data collection technique keywords listed for the years 1971–2005. Of these, 536 grants for ethnographic research were awarded by a broad array of NIH Institutes including NIDA (145), NIMH (138), NICHD (63), NINR (49), NIA (38), NCI (14), and NHLBI (8) as well as by AHRQ (19). In addition, the number of ethnographic studies (keywords: ethnography or ethnographic) funded by DHHS entities is steadily climbing with more than half funded in the last eight years (For an example, see Figure 2—Number of NIH Grants with Keywords—Ethnography or Ethnographic).

Table 3. Funding History for Qualitative Research Traditions and Strategies (CRISP Database)

Methodology Keywords	Number	Data Collection Strategy Keywords	Number
Ethnography/Ethnographic	536	Focus Group Interviews	444
Grounded Theory	121	Case Study	224
Critical/Feminist	17	Participant Observation	179
Historical Research	11	Life History	105
Metasynthesis	1	Qualitative Interviews	84
		Key Informant Interviews	60
		Oral History	11
		Guided Interviews	7

Figure 2. Number of NIH Grants with Keywords—Ethnography or Ethnographic

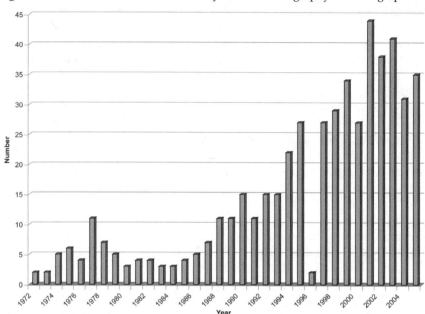

Table 4. Distinctions among NIH Grant Mechanisms

Grant Mechanism	Duration of Award (Years)	$$$ Direct Costs	Page Limits	Due Dates	Resubmit#	Renewable
R01	1–5	500 K / year with prior approval	25	2/1; 6/1; 10/1	2	Yes
R03	2	100 K	10	2/1; 6/1; 10/1	1	No
R15	3	150 K	25	1/25; 5/25; 9/25	2	Yes
R21	2	275 K	15	2/1; 6/1; 10/1	2	No
F31	1-5	Stipend + Tuition/fees	10	4/5; 8/5; 12/5	2	No

NIH Grant Mechanisms

NIH grant mechanisms include two major types: Training/Development and Research grants. Training/Development grants include F-series grants for predoctoral (F31), postdoctoral (F32), and senior scientist (F33) categories; T-series pre- and/or postdoctoral Institutional Training Grants; and K-series Career Development Awards (e.g., K01, K23). Research grant mechanisms include the R01 (Investigator-Initiated and New Investigator) as well as R03 (Small Grant), R15 (AREA), and R21 (Exploratory Development Awards). Research is also supported through the P-series awards for program project and center grants, as well as through contracts and cooperative agreements. The R01 grant mechanism constitutes the majority of applications and awards in most Institutes' portfolio of grants.

These grant mechanisms and their specific requirements change over time. In addition, Institutes within NIH vary their funding mechanisms and specifications, such as application due dates, page limits, budget restrictions, number of possible resubmissions, renewal options, accompanying materials, and eligibility criteria (see Table 4—Distinctions among NIH Grant Mechanisms). Up-to-date information can be found at the NIH website http://www.nih.gov/ and at the websites for each Institute. Regular updates on grant policies or new requests for proposals can be found in the NIH Guide, available online or via email (http://grants.nih.gov/grants/guide/listserv.htm).

RFAs and PAs

While most applications to NIH are investigator-initiated grants, priority areas for research are sometimes announced. Institutes and Centers issue special Requests for Applications (RFAs) and Program Announcements (PAs) to address specific issues, such as technological advances, health disparities, health crises, and world events. RFAs are invitations to submit research grant applications for a one-time competition on a specific topic. Generally, RFAs are financed through set-aside funds for a possible number of awards, although no minimum number of funded awards is promised. The RFA announcement specifies deviations from the normal grant application procedure (e.g., number of pages, budget limits, consortia agreements, and number of applications per university). Special ad hoc review panels are convened to evaluate proposals submitted in response to an RFA. PAs, on the other hand, are more general announcements of an Institute's or a combination of Institutes' interest in a particular research area. Unlike RFAs, PAs generally do not have set-aside funds. These grants are usually submitted on regular unsolicited application deadlines and conform to the standard PHS 398 instructions. In addition, Initial Review Groups (IRGs) typically review grants submitted in response to PAs.

NIH Grant Applications

In this section, we discuss preparation of the NIH grant application. We provide an introduction to the standard proposal format, the Public Health

Service (PHS) 398 Form (See appendix, Tips for Preparing a PHS 398 Application). We then review each area of the Research Plan including the Specific Aims, Background and Significance, Preliminary Studies, and Research Design and Methods. Lastly, we briefly discuss mock reviews and outline the procedures by which grant proposals are processed when they arrive at NIH.

The PHS 398 Form

The "PHS 398 Form" (revised 04/2006) is a less imposing document than its somber title suggests. The document comes in three sections and contains step-by-step instructions, helpful hints, and all necessary forms. The PHS 398 Instructions estimates that it takes about 40 hours to complete the application forms (excluding development of the scientific plan and the Human Subjects section). Part I of the PHS 398 is the most useful for grant applicants, containing clear instructions for preparing the application. This section begins with grant writing tips, award information, award trends, and contact information for all funding units of NIH and other relevant DHHS offices. Part I also provides links to full explanations of various types of grant mechanisms and offers suggestions for various phases of the application process. Part II contains supplemental instructions for preparing the Human Subjects section of the proposal. Part III contains policies, assurances, and definitions. The PHS 398 packet is available on the web at: http://grants.nih.gov/grants/funding/phs398/phs398.html.

Research Plan Sections

The specific points researchers must address in NIH grant proposals are straightforward. Each section of the PHS 398 application is discussed below. Italics indicate the directions from the PHS 398 Instructions followed by an interpretation of these guidelines.

Section A—Specific Aims

"List the broad, long-term objectives and the goal of the specific research proposed, e.g., to test a stated hypothesis, create a novel design, solve a specific problem, challenge an existing paradigm or clinical practice, address a critical barrier to progress in the field, or develop new technology. One page is recommended."

The specific aims section sets the stage for the entire proposal and is perhaps the most important part of the application. This section should provide an overview of the nature of the problem and its significance; a summary of the gaps in the literature; and the purpose of the project. Aims should be clear, distinct, and logically derived from the problem statement. A clear rationale for employing a qualitative approach is required and must be linked to the overall project purpose, whether it is for descriptive as with concept refinement, taxonomy generation, instrument development, sensitization, and perhaps meta-synthesis, or for more interpretive purposes.[32] For example, phenomenology may be the method of choice if the purpose is to understand the meaning of the lived experience of a given phenomena for informants; grounded theory is often selected to uncover/understand basic social processes and generate theory; ethnographers attempt to understand patterns and/or processes grounded by culture; and critical approaches are used to uncover tacit knowledge and issues of power and oppression. A common problem that applicants encounter with the study aims concerns the lack of consistency applicants maintain throughout the proposal. Reviewers need to see a clear link from each aim through data collection and data analyses.

Section B—Background and Significance

"Briefly sketch the background leading to the present application, critically evaluate existing knowledge, and specifically identify the gaps that the project is intended to fill. State concisely the importance and health relevance of the research described in this application by relating the specific aims to the broad, long-term objectives. If the aims of the application are achieved, state how scientific knowledge or clinical practice will be advanced. Describe the effect of these studies on the concepts, methods, technologies, treatments, services or preventative interventions that drive this field. Two to three pages are recommended."

The background and significance section substantiates the importance of the topic and locates the proposed study in the literature through an insightful and critical review of relevant research. This state-of-the-science review is a synthesis that specifies gaps in current knowledge and articulates how the study builds, expands, or addresses areas previously neglected or inadequately approached. The literature should be current with the majority of supporting references published within the past five years unless clearly of historical importance. Further, as scientific reviewers are drawn from a wide pool of interdisciplinary fields, so too should the supporting literature. A background section that is narrowly confined within disciplinary boundaries generally does not provide a cogent argument that stirs reviewers. In short, the literature review should be comprehensive but not exhaustive. A few recent publications offer keen insights on the background section of qualitative proposals. Penrod[11] contends that the use of a conceptual framework or theoretical orientation does not necessarily result in deductive thinking or *a priori* rigidity. Cutcliffe and Stevenson[14] provide the following recommendations for the background section of the research proposal:

1) Highlight deficiencies in our current understanding of the phenomenon;
2) Indicate the value of the proposed study (e.g., health outcomes and societal, economic, or political merits of the research);
3) Point out unique features in the proposed study that will contribute to extant science or knowledge;
4) Explain how the proposed study relates to current national priorities as well as to the mission of the Institute;

5) Envision the contributions that the proposed study will make for clinical practice; and

6) Ensure the argument is cogent, logical, and well referenced.

In the significance section, the goal is to key the reviewer into the importance of this work for the advancement of science and the betterment of the human condition. Although some qualitative traditions (e.g., grounded theory, phenomenology) require that the investigator minimize bias by limiting *a priori* knowledge of the topic, grant applicants must clearly articulate the importance of their subject matter. Significance is established by a number of strategies, including the targeted use of statistics. Though qualitative researchers may resist using statistics to substantiate their arguments, doing so limits the applicant's ability to connect with scientists who conduct quantitatively oriented investigations. Documenting the magnitude of the problem, the number of persons affected by a disease, the actual and predicted costs of treatment, or the degree of pain and suffering experienced are powerful strategies to establish significance for content experts.

Section C—Preliminary Studies

"For new applications, use this section to provide an account of the principal investigator/program director's preliminary studies pertinent to this application, including his/her preliminary experience with and outreach to the proposed racial/ethnic group members. This information will also help to establish the experience and competence of the investigator to pursue the proposed project. Except for Exploratory/Development Grants (R21/R33), Small Research Grants (R03), and Phase I Small Business Research Grants (R41/R43), peer review committees generally view preliminary data as an essential part of a research grant application. Preliminary data often aid the reviewers in assessing the likelihood of the success of the proposed project. Six to eight pages are recommended."

The preliminary studies section identifies the applicant's background, experience, and expertise for this study. Expertise may lie in formal educational preparation, language fluency, or technical skills. Specifically identify previous research with significant findings, especially from any feasibility studies using the proposed methods, setting, and population. Small project funding is often the first step in a program of research and helps prepare the investigator to write and manage larger grants.[11,33]

Section D—Research Design and Methods

"Describe the research design conceptual or clinical framework, procedures, and analyses to be used to accomplish the specific aims of the project. Unless addressed separately in Section i, include how the data will be collected, analyzed, and interpreted as well as the data-sharing plan as appropriate. Describe any new methodology and its advantage over existing methodologies. Describe any novel concepts, approaches, tools, or technologies for the proposed studies. Discuss the potential difficulties and limitations of the proposed procedures and alternative

approaches to achieve the aims. As part of this section, provide a tentative sequence or timetable for the project. Point out any procedures, situations, or materials that may be hazardous to personnel and the precautions to be exercised. Although no specific number of pages is recommended for the Research Design and Methods section, be as succinct as possible. There is no requirement that all 25 pages allotted for items A-D be used."

The research design and methods section addresses how the project will be conducted. Name and describe the methodology (e.g., descriptive qualitative, ethnographic field study, interpretive phenomenology), citing general methods resources[34-36] as well as methodological specialists.[31] A common complaint lodged against qualitative proposals in general is the overuse of disciplinary jargon. Although at least one of the three peer reviewers assigned to write a critique is typically a qualitative researcher, others may be assigned as reviewers because of their expertise in the substantive topic area (e.g., caregivers' research) or population (e.g., Mexican-Americans). A grant application is not the place for an epistemological treatise or exposition but rather for clear, straightforward language. A particular caution is to guard against inconsistencies in the terms and approaches. An example of one such inconsistency would be proposing the use of theoretical sampling and constant comparative method, but planning to collect all data before beginning the coding and analyses.

Continuously provide rationales and specific details in all portions of the research design section. In most forms of naturalistic inquiry, investigators typically use one or a combination of research strategies including participant observation, interviews, and document analysis. When using a combination of data collection or if deviating from standard approaches, explain the rationale for this decision. Although all possible scenarios cannot be controlled or prespecified for purposive sampling, recruitment, or data collection, provide information about what may happen at each of these points in the study, detailing decision logic and the benefits and limitations of a particular design compromise rather than glossing over potential problems.

Sample/Participants/Informants

Describe the setting, the rationale for selecting it, and strategies to gain entry. Identify and justify the selection of the targeted population, as well as the unit of sampling: persons, families, events, activities, or situations. Identify criteria for participant inclusion and exclusion. Explain probable procedures for identifying and recruiting participants. Becker[37] highlights the need to differentiate between selective and theoretical sampling—with selective sampling involving a calculated decision about the sampling specifications prior to beginning data collection, and theoretical sampling as an ongoing process of data collection determined by the emerging theory. Make sure that the sampling strategy selected is reflected in the criteria for participant inclusion, as well as strategies for data saturation and analysis.

A number of investigators[13,35,37-40] have identified considerations in determining the number of participants required across qualitative methods including: a) the scope of the study (the broader the study, the greater the number); b) the level of the data (deeper vs. surface levels); c) frequency of contact (longitudinal vs. single data points); d) whether the data are direct (personal) or indirect (shadowed—experiences described by others); e) the quality of the data anticipated (the better the quality, the fewer the participants); and f) whether the aim is to describe essences or dimensions (locating core or essences require fewer participants than does dimensionalizing and pattern finding). Small samples may be appropriate for homogeneous or critical case investigations. For most approaches, however, recruitment of participants (or the sampling unit) should continue until there is data redundancy or saturation.[41]

Data Collection

Each research question may require a different type of data and a different data collection strategy. Explain why each data collection strategy is needed (what kinds of data should result) and its rationale. Identify likely types of participants, settings, purposes of interaction, behaviors observed, and investigator's role. Describe anticipated strategies for data collection: where, when, with whom, and how often. If using observational techniques, also specify the anticipated types of settings or circumstances. Indicate the form of the data such as field notes or interviews (remembered only, from notes, or taped audio and/or video). If research assistants collect data, what are the criteria for selecting persons? What training will the research assistant receive initially, and what measures will be used to protect data collection from "drift?"

If conducting interviews, specify the anticipated type (individual versus group), the degree of structure, the estimated length, and the types of questions likely to be asked (at least at the initial phases). Each of these dimensions has its nuances for specification. For example, in justifying the type of interview method it may be helpful to draw on Agar and MacDonald's[42] comparison of the benefits and limitations of focus group versus individual interviews. Or in explaining group interviews, Coreil[43] provides a useful continuum of four types of group interviews (ranging from the most structured consensus panel to focus groups to natural groups to community interviews) with distinguishing features and limitations of each. In addition, discuss the most likely process interviewers will keep for making notes (e.g., date, circumstance, problems, or field facilitations, as well as a personal journal detailing emotions, feelings, and/or insights).

Data Processing and Analysis

All phases of data processing should be anticipated, including likely forms of the data, the structuring strategies, and coding schemes. For example, how will interview data be processed? Will they be taped? Will they be transcribed and by whom? Will interviews be verified for accuracy of transcription? Data processing and analysis often begin soon after initial data collection. If this is not the case in the proposed study, offer a reason. If using a computer program to sort and merge data, explain the rationale for its selection and anticipated uses in this study. Demonstrate expertise with qualitative analysis software by illustrating data management in prior efforts.

Methods for data coding and analysis are continually evolving and need clarification in the research proposal. The numerous terms used for similar activities and the lack of consistency in the definitions and use of terms must be addressed. Proposals should indicate whether the coding and analysis will be conducted at a descriptive and/or interpretive level. Then, specific details of anticipated coding procedures should be presented. What will be coded—whole text or discrete sections? Will coding use an open style or a partial or complete template? Will any potential codes or coding frames come from the literature or prior work? If new codes are generated, will previously coded transcripts be re-coded? For each topic, describe levels of structure and different types of coding requirements.[44]

Rigor

While rigor for quantitative research is assessed by relatively well-defined criteria, varied types of criteria are used for qualitative studies. Some qualitative investigators use the terms reliability and validity and some oppose the use of those terms.[45-51] Regardless of preferences in terminology, it is important to detail a section on rigor and quality control, clearly defining the various strategies used. These strategies vary widely across and within approaches.[2,20,35,41,52-68]

The role of the investigator should also be explicitly described. This description goes well beyond the idea of "the investigator as instrument" and addresses assumptions regarding the method and the implications of potential sources of investigator bias. While phenomenologists are usually most clear about identifying investigator biases in working through issues for bracketing, all investigators should address this issue even when they do not use this term.

Mock Review

The strength of the research plan plays a major role in determining whether a grant proposal is considered credible and fundable by its reviewers. Cohen, Knafl, and Dzurec[12] reviewed nineteen NIH grant application summary statements (i.e., "pink sheets") from 1986–1990. Applications with very good scores shared major strengths: the aims were clear and logical; strong literature reviews were provided; all had an important topic and designs consistent with aims; and most built on previous work. Priority scores indicating less good (over 200) scores tended to have an inadequate, unfocused literature review; biased, inappropriate or unclear sampling technique; lacking or insufficient rationale for sample size; and inadequate specification of a data analysis plan.[12]

Therefore, before submitting a proposal, applicants might conduct a "mock review" using NIH review criteria to assess the proposal's overall merits and problematic aspects. In planning for an internal review, allow several months to write, rewrite, format, and review the document. Next, schedule a mock review with colleagues who are successful grant applicants. The mock review process may also offer junior faculty and graduate students an opportunity to hone their review skills. A reviewer who is unfamiliar with qualitative methods or outside the field of expertise is often able to spot "gaps," confusing terms, and defensive or pejorative phrasing. Finally, take the suggestions of peer reviewers seriously and make thoughtful revisions based upon the scientific soundness of their advice.

Processing Grant Proposals

At the time of submission, attach a cover letter to the proposal if requesting assignment (for funding) to a specific Institute, as well as referral (for review) to a particular Scientific Review Group (SRG). Once submitted, most NIH grants move through the centralized Center for Scientific Review (CSR) where intake personnel read the abstract and assign the grant to an Institute as well as to a particular SRG. The SRG (sometimes referred to as "study sections") is the peer review group that will score the proposal. Two major types of SRGs exist: Initial Review Groups, or standing panels that review most investigator-initiated grants and most applications in response to PAs; and Special Emphasis Panels, or ad hoc groups most often convened for reviewing special mechanisms (e.g., RFAs) or to eliminate a conflict of interest (e.g., the PI serves on the Initial Review Group that would otherwise review the proposal).

Once the proposal is processed through the CSR, the principal investigator receives a confirmation notice (Assignment Notification) through the NIH Electronic Research Administration website (or, eRA Commons). After receiving this notice of assignment, check the roster of the appointed members on that review panel. Investigators may wish to contact the Scientific Review Administrator (indicated on the Assignment Notification) if there are concerns about the potential reviewers (e.g., a particular area of expertise needed for review of your application or a conflict of interest that might not be apparent). While most study sections that review social and behavioral research contain members with qualitative research expertise, a researcher may request a particular kind of expertise if it is not readily identifiable on the roster. Researchers should *never* contact members of the Scientific Review Group concerning an application.

Peer Review Process at NIH

The policies, review criteria, and instructions for peer review panel members are public documents located at: http://www.csr.nih.gov/welcome.htm. Review criteria were modified extensively in 1997, again in October 2004. The 1997 version was changed to make criteria more relevant to clinical, translational, and interdisciplinary research as outlined by the NIH Roadmap (see http://nihroadmap.nih.gov/ for more details). The current five criteria for evaluation are listed below in *italics* and include: significance, approach, innovation, investigator, and environment.[69] The updated criteria also emphasize that the relative weight of each criterion may vary across applications, and that an application "need not be strong in all categories to be judged likely to have a major scientific impact." Below each area of evaluation, relevant points for qualitative proposals are noted.

Significance

Does this study address an important problem? If the aims of the application are achieved, how will scientific knowledge or clinical practice be advanced? What will be the effect of these studies on the concepts, methods, technologies, treatments, services, or preventative interventions that drive this field?

Reviewers are now asked to consider both the value of a research proposal from a basic science perspective as well as the practical applicability of the study results. Applicants should clearly identify the significance of the proposal in the abstract, aims, and the background sections. In order to maintain consistency of vision, the significance statement and the specific aims may be repeated verbatim throughout the proposal.

Approach

Are the conceptual or clinical framework, design, methods, and analyses adequately developed, well-integrated, well-reasoned, and appropriate to the aims of the project? Does the applicant acknowledge potential problem areas and consider alternative tactics?

The approach criterion assesses how the research design of the proposed project fits within the overall state of the science. In conducting an evaluation of the approach, reviewers consider all sections of the research plan, with particular emphasis on Section D: Research Design. A conceptual framework may also be evaluated in this section. Reviewers will evaluate the proposed involvement of human/animal subjects, as well as the plan for inclusion of minorities and members of both sexes/genders. Reviewers factor these components together to provide a summary score for the scientific and technical merit of the application. Researchers who propose the use of qualitative methods must make the strongest argument possible for their approach, selecting scientific techniques to best answer the research question, rather than choosing methods based upon personal preferences. Qualitative approaches are more obviously useful early in a new area of science; their application may be considered less appropriate as the area is more developed.

Innovation

Is the project original and innovative? For example: Does the project challenge existing paradigms or clinical practice; address an innovative hypothesis or critical barrier to progress in the field? Does the project develop or employ novel concepts, approaches or methodologies, tools, or technologies for this area?

The applicant must demonstrate creative thinking and the application of novel concepts in their proposals. Reviewers are asked whether an application is the "first ever" or "first to use" project to incorporate the proposed concepts, methods, or technologies. For example, in the funded R01 project, *Analytic Techniques for Qualitative Metasynthesis,* Sandelowski was the first researcher who was funded using a method of integrating findings from multiple qualitative studies.[70]

Investigator

Are the investigators appropriately trained and well suited to carry out this work? Is the work proposed appropriate to the experience level of the principal investigator and other researchers? Does the investigative team bring complementary and integrated expertise to the project (if applicable)?

The investigator criterion addresses the competencies of both the principal investigator and the research team. Expertise is evaluated by the history of training and publications. The application should contain evidence that needed expertise—substantive, methodological, and technical—is available on the team for each component of the research design. Expertise that is specific rather than general is necessary. If an applicant has never used an analytic strategy or data collection technique, collaboration with experienced consultants can mitigate this lack of expertise.

Environment

Does the scientific environment in which the work will be done contribute to the probability of success? Do the proposed studies benefit from unique features of the scientific environment, or subject populations, or employ useful collaborative arrangements? Is there evidence of institutional support?

Reviewers consider the adequacy of the institutional and research environments as support structures for the proposed study. Items regarded include the research intensity of the institution, computer/technological resources, libraries/databases, and the availability of space necessary for the proposed research, as well as interdepartmental consideration.

Summary Statements

After peer review, the investigator accesses the summary statement (sometimes called "pink sheets") via the eRA Commons on the NIH website at https://commons.era.nih.gov/commons/. The summary statement includes the proposal's priority score; determination of the acceptability of the human/animal subjects protections and recruitment plans; a summary of the reviewers' discussion; and detailed reviewer critiques. The summary statement does not indicate whether or not the grant will be funded; it does, however, offer considerable information about how the proposal was received by its initial reviewers. The researcher may wish to contact the program officer (indicated on the summary statement) to clarify reviewers'

Summary Points

- There is growing recognition within NIH that qualitative and community-based participatory methods are particularly useful for addressing health care quality and system change issues.
- Prospective applicants should know as much as possible about an Institute's mission, interests, and goals and ensure that the proposed research is closely aligned with the Institute's strategic plans and areas of program emphasis.
- Grant applications should provide a clear rationale for employing a qualitative approach, establish consistent links from each aim to data collection and data analyses, and avoid overuse of disciplinary jargon.
- Specific strategies for ensuring scientific rigor must be clearly defined and described.
- Proposals on important topics that are carefully conceived, meticulously planned, and well-written can use ethnographic, phenomenological, or community-based participatory research methods *and* obtain substantial grant awards.

---

comments, to interpret the percentile score, or to obtain guidance on resubmitting the application.

Conclusion

In this chapter we have discussed specific strategies for obtaining funding for aging-related studies using qualitative research methods. Through an overview of the structure, organization, and processes of the DHHS, we have shown that many Institutes and Centers within the NIH have a long history of supporting scientists with programs of research that are person-centered, innovative in their solutions to health disparities in elder populations, and pioneering in their models to address dysfunctional systems of care. Proposals on important topics that are carefully conceived, meticulously planned, and well-written can use ethnographic, phenomenological, or community-based participatory research methods *and* obtain substantial grant awards. Investigators using qualitative methodologies can maximize the likelihood that their research proposals will achieve competitive priority scores by adhering to the principles itemized in this chapter. Finally, it is important to address problems that are significant in the lives of older adults. Select research *approaches* that are well-reasoned and appropriate to the aims of the project. Be *innovative* in the conceptualization and execution of the study. Gather a team of *investigators* who are dynamic, creative, and dedicated to improving the health of older adults through the advancement of scientific knowledge. And work in supportive and stimulating *environments* that contribute to the probability of the researchers' success. Write grants often and rewrite them as necessary. Experience proves to be the best teacher of all.

References

1) Jones, R. Why Do Qualitative Research? *British Medical Journal.* 1995; 311: 2.
2) Popay, J., Rogers, A., and Williams, G. Rationale and Standards for the Systematic Review of Qualitative Literature in Health Services Research. *Qualitative Health Research.* 1998; 8: 341-351.
3) Shortell, S.M. The Emergence of Qualitative Methods in Health Services Research. *Health Services Research.* 1999; 34: 1083-1089.
4) Pope, C., van Royen, P., and Baker, R. Qualitative Methods in Research on Healthcare Quality. *Quality and Safety in Health Care.* 2002, 11: 148-152.
5) Tripp-Reimer, T., Doebbeling, B. Qualitative Perspectives in Translational Research. *Worldviews on Evidence-Based Nursing.* 2004; 1: S65-S72.
6) Tripp-Reimer, T., Choi, E., Kelley, L.S., and Enslein, J. Cultural Barriers to Care: Inverting the Problem. *Diabetes Spectrum.* 2001; 14: 13-22.
7) Morse, J.M. Learning to Drive from a Manual? *Qualitative Health Research.* 1997; 7: 181-183.
8) Tripp-Reimer, T. Health Heritage Project: A Research Proposal Submitted to the Division of Nursing. *Western Journal of Nursing Research.* 1986; 8: 207-224.
9) Tripp-Reimer T, Cohen M. Funding Strategies for Qualitative Research. In Morse J. (Ed.). *Qualitative Research: A Contemporary Dialogue.* Rockville, MD: Aspen, 1989, pp. 225-238.
10) Carey, M.A. and Swanson, J. Funding for Qualitative Research. *Qualitative Health Research.* 2003; 13: 852-856.
11) Penrod, J. Getting Funded: Writing a Successful Qualitative Small-Project Proposal. *Qualitative Health Research.* 2003; 13: 821-832.
12) Cohen, M.Z., Knafl, K., and Dzurec, L.C. Grant Writing for Qualitative Research. *IMAGE: Journal of Nursing Scholarship.* 1993; 25: 151-156.
13) Kuzel, A.J. Sampling in Qualitative Inquiry. In Crabtree, B.F. and Miller, W.L. (Eds.). *Doing Qualitative Research.* Newbury Park: Sage Publications, 1992, pp. 31-44.
14) Cutcliffe, J. and Stevenson, C. The Long And Winding Road: Obtaining Funding for Qualitative Research Proposals. *Nurse Researcher.* 2001; 9: 52-62.
15) Sandelowski, M., Davis, D.H., and Harris, B.G. Artful Design: Writing the Proposal for Research in the Naturalist Paradigm. *Research in Nursing and Health.* 1989; 12: 77-84.
16) Roth, W-M. Evaluation and Adjudication of Research Proposals: Vagaries and Politics of Funding. *Forum: Qualitative Social Research* [serial online]. September 2002; 3(3). Available at: http://www.qualitative-research.net/fqs-texte/3-02/3-02roth-e.htm
17) Anderson, N.B. Integrating Behavioral and Social Sciences Research at the National Institutes of Health, U.S.A. *Social Science and Medicine* 1997; 44: 1069-1071.
18) Lambert, E.Y., Ashery RS, Needle R.H. (Eds.). *Qualitative Methods in Drug Abuse and HIV Research.* (NIDA Research Monograph 157, *NIH Publication # 95-4025*). Washington, DC: National Institutes of Health, 1995.
19) Qualitative Methods in Health Services Research. Agency for Healthcare Research and Quality. Available at http://www.ahrq.gov/about/cods/cod-squal.htm
20) Devers, K.J. How Will We Know "Good" Qualitative Research When We See It? Beginning the Dialogue in Health Services Research. *Health Services Research.* 1999; 34: 1153-1188.

21) Office of Behavioral and Social Sciences Research. *Qualitative Methods in Health Research: Opportunities and Considerations in Application and Review.* Washington, DC: National Institutes of Health, 1999. Available at http://obssr.od.nih.gov/Publications/Qualitative.pdf

22) Symposium and Working Group on New Directions in Adherence Research: Using Qualitative Methods to Promote Self-Care in Diverse Populations. Available at http://obssr.od.nih.gov/Conf_Wkshp/Adherence/Qualitative_Methods.htm. (Accessed March 15, 2005.)

23) NIH Summer Institute: The Design and Conduct of Qualitative and Mixed-Method Research in Social Work and Other Health Professions. Available at http://obssr.od.nih.gov/conf_wkshp/sw/

24) Workshop on Scientific Foundations of Qualitative Research. Available at http://www.nsf.gov/pubs/2004/nsf04219/start.htm

25) National Institute on Aging. Available at http://www.nia.nih.gov/AboutNIA/

26) About the National Institute of Nursing Research. Available at http://ninr.nih.gov/ninr/research/diversity/mission.html

27) Institute of Medicine. *Crossing The Quality Chasm: A New Health Care System for the 21st Century.* Washington, DC: Institute of Medicine Committee on Quality Health Care in America, 2001.

28) Smedley, B.D., Stith, A.Y., and Nelson, A.R. (Eds.). *Unequal Treatment: Confronting Racial and Ethnic Disparities in Health Care.* Washington, DC: Institute of Medicine Committee on Understanding and Eliminating Racial and Ethnic Disparities in Health Care, 2003.

29) Fact Sheet on Racial Health Disparities. Available at http://www.clintonfoundation.org/legacy/022198-fact-sheet-on-racial-health-disparities.htm

30) Gilgun, J.F. Conjecturse and Refutations: Governmental Funding and Qualitative Research. *Qualitative Social Work,* 2002; 1: 359-375.

31) Glaser, B.G. and Strauss, A.L. *The Discovery of Grounded Theory: Strategies for Qualitative Research.* Hawthorne, NY: Aldine, 1967.

32) Knafl, K.A. and Howard, M.J. Interpreting and Reporting Qualitative Research. *Research in Nursing and Health.* 1984; 7: 17-24.

33) Morse, J.M. The Pertinence of Pilot Studies. *Qualitative Health Research.* 2003a; 7: 323-324.

34) Miles, M.B. and Huberman, A.M. *Qualitative Data Analysis: A Sourcebook of New Methods.* Beverly Hills, CA: Sage Publications, 1984.

35) Patton, M.Q. *Qualitative Evaluation and Research Methods* (2nd ed.). Newbury Park, CA: Sage Publications, 1990.

36) Tripp-Reimer, T. and Kelley, L. Qualitative Research. In Fitzpatrick, J. (Ed.). *Encyclopedia of Nursing Research.* Newbury Park, CA: Sage Publications, 1998.

37) Becker, P.H. Common Pitfalls in Published Grounded Theory Research. *Qualitative Health Research.* 1993; 3: 254-260.

38) Sandelowski, M. Focus on Qualitative Methods: Sample Size in Qualitative Research. *Research in Nursing and Health.* 1995; 18: 179-183.

39) Morse, J.M. On the Evaluation of Qualitative Proposals. *Qualitative Health Research.* 1991; 1: 147-151.

40) Morse, J.M. Determining Sample Size. *Qualitative Health Research.* 2000; 10: 3-5.

41) Lincoln, Y.S., Guba, E.G. *Naturalistic Inquiry.* Beverly Hills, CA: Sage, 1985.

42) Agar, M. and MacDonald, J. Focus Groups and Ethnography. *Human Organization.* 1995; 54: 78-86.

43) Coreil, J. Group Interview Methods in Community Health Research. *Medical Anthropology,* 1995; 16: 193-210.

44) Crabtree, B.F., William, L., and Miller, W.L. *Doing Qualitative Research*. Newbury Park: Sage Publications, 1992.

45) Beck, C.T. Reliability and Validity Issues in Phenomenological Research. *Western Journal of Nursing Research*. 1994; 16: 254-267.

46) Imle, M.A. and Atwood, J.R. Retaining Qualitative Validity While Gaining Quantitative Reliability and Validity: Development of the Transition to Parenthood Concerns Scale. *Advances in Nursing Science*. 1988; 11: 61-75.

47) Kirk, J. and Miller, M.L. *Reliability and Validity in Qualitative Research*. Beverly Hills: Sage Publications, 1986.

48) Morse, J.M. Myth #93: Reliability and Validity are not Relevant to Qualitative Inquiry. *Qualitative Health Research*. 1999; 9: 717-718.

49) Richards, L. Rigorous, Rapid, Reliable and Qualitative? Computing in Qualitative Method. *American Journal of Health Behavior*. 2002; 26: 425-430.

50) Tripp-Reimer, T. Issues of Accuracy in Qualitative Research. *Western Journal of Nursing Research,* 1984; 6: 353-355.

51) Tripp-Reimer, T. Reliability Issues in Cross-Cultural Research. *Western Journal of Nursing Research*. 1985; 7: 391-392.

52) Bruyn, S.T. *The Human Perspective in Sociology: The Methodology of Participant Observation*. Englewood Cliffs: Prentice-Hall, 1966.

53) Cobb, A.K. and Hagemaster, J.N. Ten Criteria for Evaluating Qualitative Research Proposals. *Journal of Nursing Education*. 1987; 26: 138-143.

54) Holkup, P., Tripp-Reimer, T., Salois, E., and Weinert, C. Community Based Participatory Research: An Approach to Intervention Research with Native American Communities. *Advances in Nursing Science*. 2004; 27: 162-175.

55) Hutchinson, S. and Wilson, H.S. Validity Threats in Scheduled Semistructured Research Interviews. *Nursing Research*. 1992; 41: 117-119.

56) Leininger, M.M. *Qualitative Research Methods in Nursing*. New York: Grune and Stratton, 1985.

57) Malterud, K. Qualitative Research: Standards, Challenges, and Guidelines. *The Lancet*. 2001; 358: 483-488.

58) Miles, M.B. and Huberman, A.M. (Eds.). *Qualitative Data Analysis: An Expanded Sourcebook* (2nd ed.). Thousand Oaks, CA: Sage Publications, 1994.

59) Miller, W.L. and Crabtree, B.F. Clinical Research. In Denzil, N.K. and Lincoln, Y.S. (Eds.). *Strategies of Qualitative Inquiry*. Thousand Oaks, CA: Sage Publications, 2003, pp. 397-434.

60) Morgan, D.L. Why Things (Sometimes) Go Wrong in Focus Groups. *Qualitative Health Research*. 1995; 5: 516-523.

61) Morse, J.M. A Review Committee's Guide for Evaluating Qualitative Proposals. *Qualitative Health Research*. 2003b; 13: 833-851.

62) Patton, M.Q. Enhancing the Quality and Credibility of Qualitative Analysis. *Health Services Research*. 1999; 34: 1189-1208.

63) Peck, E., Secker, J. Quality Criteria from Qualitative Research: Does Context Make a Difference? *Qualitative Health Research*. 1999; 9: 552-558.

64) Ratcliff, D. Evaluating Ethnographic Research: 5 Attributes and 12 Components. Adapted and expanded from Goetz, J.P. and LeCompte, M.D. (Eds.). *Ethnography and Qualitative Design*. Orlando, FL: Academic Press, 2002, pp. 232-243.

65) Rodgers, B.L. and Cowles, K.V. The Qualitative Research Audit Trail: A Complex Collection of Documentation. *Research in Nursing and Health*. 1993; 16: 219-226.

66) Sandelowski, M. The Problem in Rigor in Qualitative Research. *Advances in Nursing Science*. 1986; 8: 27-37.

67) Thorne, S. The Art (and Science) of Critiquing Qualitative Research. In Morse, J.M. (Ed.). *Completing a Qualitative Project: Details and Dialogue.* Thousand Oaks, CA: Sage Publications, 1997, pp. 117-132.

68) Wilson, H.S. and Hutchinson, S.A. Methodologic Mistakes in Grounded Theory. *Nursing Research.* 1996; 45: 122-124.

69) National Institute of Mental Health. *NIMH Reviewers' Critique Guide (R01).* Washington, DC: National Institutes of Health, 1993.

70) Sandelowski, M.J. *Analytic Techniques for Qualitative Metasynthesis (R01).* Washington, DC: National Institutes of Health, 2000.

Appendix for Chapter 11
Tips for Preparing a PHS 398 Application

Pay attention to formatting instructions, as well as page limitations, for a particular type of application. If these are not followed, your application will be returned to you without review.

FONT
- Use 11 point Arial or Helvetica
- Black ink and readily legible
- Exceptions: smaller type for figures, legends, graphs, charts and tables

MARGINS
- Use 8 ½" x 11" paper
- Instructions indicate ½ inch margins
- A 1 inch margin is easier for reviewers

PAGING
- Single sided and single spaced
- Number consecutively; no 11a or 14b

PHOTOS/IMAGES
- Images must be printed directly on the application page in the body of the text

COPIES
- Include original and 5 exact copies
- NO photo reduction allowed

LANGUAGE
- English only
- Avoid jargon
- Define conceptual/technical terms
- Abbreviations are acceptable— first time term is used, spell out the entire phrase and note appropriate abbreviation

GRANT TITLE
- 81 typewriter spaces (not characters)

HUMAN SUBJECTS
- You must follow all instructions in this section completely. Reviewers read this carefully and failure to address all points can be detrimental to your application.

BIOSKETCHES
- Need biosketches completed in defined NIH format from investigators and consultants

BUDGET
- Even if you think you will be using the modular budget process, make sure you complete a detailed budget.
- Use a spreadsheet program to enter every possible expense in detail.
- This practice gives you a better idea of how much it will cost to complete your proposed project.
- If you don't use the modular budget, the spreadsheet details are useful in writing the budget justification.

LETTERS OF SUPPORT
- You must have letters from consultants outlining exactly their commitment to and responsibilities in this study

- If you are using multiple data collection sites, obtain letters of support from those sites indicating willingness to participate. Such letters serve to reinforce the fact that you have thought through what you will do and where you will do it, and at least have the support of your sites.

SUBCONTRACTS

- If a multi-site grant, with work being done by investigators at other institutions, remember that you will be issuing subcontracts for this work.
- Obtain detailed (not modular) budgets and budget justifications from the investigator(s) at subcontract sites.
- Obtain appropriate letters from the institutional official agreeing to accept a subcontract if the application is funded.

Chapter 12

Qualitative Research in Gerontology: Preparing a Credible and Publishable Manuscript

Sara A. Quandt, PhD

Introduction: The Challenges

Investigators who publish qualitative research in gerontology begin with the knowledge that the majority of published work in the field is based on quantitative, rather than qualitative, data. With few deviations, published manuscripts based on quantitative data follow a standard formula of introduction, background, methods, results, and conclusions. This familiar template provides a comfortable structure and direction to both novice and seasoned authors. It is the standard many editors and reviewers use to judge submitted manuscripts. This expectation poses a challenge for authors of research reports based on qualitative research: because their manuscripts do not often fit this mold, they may appear anomalous to many reviewers and editors alike. Therefore, the likelihood of having a qualitative paper accepted is unfortunately reduced.

A second challenge is that many researchers conducting qualitative research today have not been educated in the epistemology of qualitative work that has been a long tradition in a limited number of disciplines, such as anthropology and sociology. Thus these researchers may not have read widely enough in qualitative research to get a strong sense of how qualitative research should be written for publication.

A final challenge is that as qualitative research is now being adopted by such applied disciplines as medicine, public health, and nursing, these researchers are seeking to publish their work in journals to which this work is foreign.

This chapter will address these challenges by providing a step-by-step approach to publishing qualitative research in aging. The process begins with choosing a target journal, continues with crafting the manuscript, and finishes with taking the manuscript through the peer-review process. While the discussion of preparing and publishing qualitative research will be tailored to publishing in gerontology, the steps are easily transferable to other areas of public health research.

Choosing a Journal

It's a fact: only a small proportion of the thousands of health and behavior-related journals published ever contain papers based on qualitative research.

That means that the first task for prospective authors is to do their *own* research to find a journal that is appropriate for publishing the manuscripts they intend to write. Exploring the suitability of potential journals for publishing qualitative research should start early in the process. Ideally, the search should start when one reviews the literature to plan a research study. The researcher will note the different types of qualitative research and learn the kind of research each journal publishes. Does the journal contain articles that are long, ethnographic pieces with rich description? Or are these articles more concise summaries of qualitative research that emphasize ideas contained in the qualitative material, but present little of the actual data? The results of this search will give the prospective author a good idea of the publication possibilities of each journal.

Choosing a journal starts in earnest when the research is complete and a publication is planned. While it is possible to write a manuscript and then search for a journal, it is probably more efficient to have a specific journal in mind before designing the manuscript. It is helpful to start by making a list of journals that fit the audience for the research. While knowing where key previous studies have been published is a start, it is also helpful to consider a wide range of journals before making a firm decision to target a manuscript to a specific journal.

Journals can fall into several categories. Some journals have a methodological focus. For example, *Qualitative Health Research* and *Qualitative Sociology* restrict their papers to only those that use qualitative methods. Other journals have a disease focus. Some examples of this kind are *Diabetes Care, Arthritis Care & Research,* and *Cancer.* Other journals target research on a specific population or population segment, such as the *Journal of Rural Health, Journal of Immigrant Health,* and *Hispanic Journal of Behavioral Science.* Some take a disciplinary focus. Some journals of this type include *Western Journal of Nursing Research* and *Medical Anthropology Quarterly.* Of particular interest to gerontologists are those that take an aging focus. Some of these are the *Journal of Gerontology,* the *Gerontologist,* and the *Journal of the American Geriatrics Society.* Finally, there are general health or medical journals, such as the *American Journal of Public Health, Journal of the American Medical Association,* and *Lancet.* The list of possible journals that a qualitative researcher should consider is likely to include journals from different categories.

The next step is to find out if the journals of interest currently welcome qualitative research. Internet resources available today have made this step easier for authors. A researcher should check the table of contents of recent issues to see whether qualitative research has been included. It should be noted that journals with only an occasional qualitative paper may only include such research as part of a special issue, or those qualitative papers may have had some other privileged route to publication. It is important furthermore to make sure that qualitative research has been published under the *current* editor, as editorial policies can and do change with the preferences and background of each editor. Names on the current editorial board provide useful information. If there are no researchers with qualitative expertise included on the editorial board, it is unlikely that the journal has a serious commitment to reviewing qualitative research. The mission statement for the journal is also significant. Does it specifically mention publishing qualitative research as a goal of the journal?

After narrowing the list of possible journals, it is a good idea for an author to gather his or her own qualitative data about publishing. Asking mentors who publish qualitative data about their experiences with different journals can provide insight into the pros and cons of a specific journal, as well as open up new possibilities that may not be on the original list of journals.

Who is the intended reader for the proposed article? Besides choosing a journal open to qualitative research, an author needs to think about the intended audience for the paper. Readers have specific and varied expectations. Basic researchers, for example, will expect to see something different than might be expected by practitioners. The latter will be most interested in practical applications of the research. Specialists will expect the writing to focus on their particular field more than will generalists. It is vital that the intended audience of the journal is congruent with the content of the paper to be submitted. Michael Cheang, for example, published a paper in *Journal of Aging Studies* interpreting the practice of older adults' congregating in fast food restaurants as important for their ability to create a place other than work or home for social interaction and "play"[1]. The paper fits this journal with its applications only implied. Had it been written for a more applied journal such as *The Gerontologist*, the author would have needed to include more direct suggestions for social workers or activities directors on how to help older adults to create such a beneficial social gathering place.

The final step is to review the "Instructions for Authors" from a recent journal or the journal's website. The instructions provide structure and set limits on manuscripts submitted to the journal. Page and word limits are of primary importance to many qualitative researchers. Journals vary widely on such limits and on what is included in these limits. For example, *Qualitative Health Research* currently has no page limits, but the journal cautions authors that their "manuscripts must be 'tight' and as long as they need to be." *Journal of Aging Studies* also states no limits on number of pages. Despite the policies of these two journals, most others are explicit about the maximum length of manuscripts. Some journals count references, while others only count text. Although some journals count the words included in tables and figures, most of them do not. Because the data for qualitative research are often integrated into the text rather than presented in tables, qualitative authors may be at a disadvantage in presenting supporting data. Some journals recognize this important difference between methodological orientations. For example, *The Journals of Gerontology: Social Science* currently includes in their instructions to authors the statement: "Articles using qualitative methodology must be concisely written, but may require somewhat greater length." However, this accommodation to qualitative reporting is rare. In considering page limits, authors should know that reviewers often request that more information be added to the manuscript, and that editors frequently ask that the final version of a manuscript be shortened to a length even less than the published limits.

Choosing a journal that fits the research conducted, the intended audience, and the length and style of paper that a qualitative researcher intends to write is an important first step in the process of preparing a manuscript for publication. Time spent carefully considering the issues raised here will raise the probability of acceptance of the manuscript. Once a target journal is chosen and the manuscript structure and limits imposed by the journal are known, the author is ready to write the paper.

Crafting the Manuscript

Each manuscript should have a minimum set of components. While they do not have to be labeled as such, there needs to be a problem statement, a conceptual framework, a description of methods, a report of findings, and a discussion of what the findings mean. Unlike the author of a paper on quantitative research, the qualitative author is usually armed with considerable text when the process of writing the manuscript begins. This text includes field notes, interview transcripts, and other text. The key is to move from this existing text to a self-contained manuscript.

Stating the Problem and Purpose

In order to start the paper, the clearest point of departure is to develop a succinct declaration of the problem or question the research addresses and to define the purpose of the particular paper being presented. The problem statement should be no more than a couple of paragraphs, and it should clearly lay out the need for the study. In most cases, investigators describe a shortcoming of the existing literature and situate the new paper as addressing this gap or problem. In other cases, the objective of the proposed paper may arise from unmet needs of the population in question.

Because qualitative research produces a wealth of information and ideas, it is crucial to focus on a manageable goal for the paper. It is helpful to summarize the purpose of the study that will be addressed in the paper in a single sentence. This sentence will help keep the content of the paper manageable and will provide a focal point by which to evaluate how the ideas and text fit into the paper as it is being written.

In the purpose statement, it is helpful to use words that convey to the reader the qualitative approach taken in the research. Creswell[2] suggests encoding the problem statement with words that convey to the reader the particular tradition of inquiry from which the study arises. For example, a grounded theory study might use words such as "generate" or "develop," while an ethnographic study would be more likely to use words like "cultural theme," and a phenomenological study might talk about "experience," "meaning," and "description." The use of such words signals to the reader what the final products of the study will be.

Grounding the Research

Having written a problem statement, writers use the review of the literature to elaborate on the statement. This review has two purposes. The first is to make clear the theoretical foundation or conceptual framework that guides the study. The second is to summarize the studies in the literature germane to the current study. Furthermore, this review should uncover the contradictions or gaps in the current research that the study is intended to address. One important and common mistake that qualitative researchers make is to review only the qualitative research on a topic. This focus implies that the existing quantitative literature has no bearing on qualitative research. This position is difficult to defend and will cause reviewers with expertise in the topic to be highly skeptical of the literature review's thoroughness.

As both qualitative and quantitative research contribute to an understanding of a particular phenomenon, the relevant literature of each approach should be reviewed in the paper. For example, in an ethnographic study of older rural adults' interpretation and management of hunger and food insufficiency, Quandt and colleagues[3] drew upon an earlier survey in rural Appalachia[4] which had suggested that a series of "belt-tightening" behaviors would be undertaken before government safety net programs like food stamps would be used. This quantitative survey predicted not only the order of food-related behaviors, but also the attitudes these older adults might hold toward not having enough food. Such quantitative data provided a good place to start for a qualitative study to explore people's attitudes toward food insecurity and acceptable ways of dealing with it in rural communities.

Similarly, Mitteness and Barker situated their mixed-method study of the meaning and management of urinary incontinence in older adults in the shortcomings of the epidemiologic literature on the prevalence and treatment of the condition.[5,6] By showing the high prevalence of the condition juxtaposed with the prevailing medical opinion that the condition is treatable, these researchers set the stage for their findings that American society stigmatizes incontinent adults as incompetent. In this way, the researchers helped explain the extraordinary measures elders take to hide or personally manage their condition.

By effectively grounding the research in the literature previously published, a qualitative researcher creates a "need" for the paper. This lets readers know why they should read further and helps them situate the research findings within what else is known about the topic.

Describing Procedures

The next section of a manuscript describes the study's methods and presents a rationale for why these methods were chosen. This section is important because it allows the reviewer and other readers to evaluate the quality of the work to be presented. Ironically, it is the section perhaps the most often underdeveloped in qualitative manuscripts.

The section needs to describe data collection methods used. It is important to include why qualitative methods were used for the data collection in the study. Because different research questions can require different methods, reviewers expect to be assured that the researcher has chosen the best method, given the problem being investigated. The particular data collection technique should be described and justified. It is important to explain that the researcher has made a deliberate and informed choice of the best methods to use. For example, it should be clear that a researcher did not use focus groups simply because he or she has expertise in that type of data collection. Thus, reviewers will want to know the rationale if focus groups were used in a research project involving frail older persons. They may need to be convinced of the suitability of this method because focus groups typically exclude home-bound persons and present problems for those with hearing loss and other communication disorders.

The description and the rationale for the sampling strategy are also important to include. The sampling strategy must fit the problem to be addressed. For example, drawing a sample from senior centers is appropriate when the goal is to evaluate the health beliefs of senior center participants. However, because of differential senior center participation, using senior centers as a sampling frame is likely to be perceived as biased if the goal is to evaluate the health beliefs of *all* older adults in a community.

As part of the sampling strategy, it is also advisable to list inclusion and exclusion criteria for participation and describe recruitment procedures. These criteria should be reasonable for the problem under investigation. Unlike most quantitative research which generally relies on random sampling, qualitative research rarely uses random selection. The researcher should be sure to state why a randomized approach was not used, even though the rationale is obvious to a qualitative researcher. It can be pointed out that some data are often best gained through a key informant or through carefully selected representatives of key groups because knowledge in a community is differentially distributed among community members. This idea may not be familiar to all readers. It is also worth pointing out the seemingly obvious fact that a qualitative respondent must be articulate enough and willing to talk in order to provide data. Recruitment procedures should be described. In addition, many journals want to have assurance that the recruitment strategy was approved by the Institutional Review Board (IRB). The steps and choices should be articulated clearly.

It is also necessary to include a rationale for the sample size used in the research. Quantitative reviewers may be accustomed to seeing a power analysis to justify the sample size. While such an analysis is not possible or appropriate in qualitative research, the reader of a qualitative paper deserves assurances that sufficient numbers of persons participated to allow one to trust the conclusions. For example, if the study goal is to capture the *range* of ideas about a topic, sampling until saturation is reached (that is, no new information is being provided by respondents) is an appropriate explanation. Strategies used to determine that sufficient numbers of persons were included should be described.

Data analysis should be described in enough detail that a reader knows what was done. As in quantitative research, it is not enough to say that one used a particular software program. The steps should be presented in sequence in the paper so the reader can visualize the process that was undertaken from the raw data to the conclusions. Because qualitative software programs are primarily organizational tools and do not actually perform analysis in the sense that statistical software does, description of software can be misunderstood by non-qualitative reviewers who will expect numeric results. Because qualitative data analysis does not have the equivalent of a statistical p-value to assure that a result is not due to chance, it is important to provide detail that will assure the reader that steps have been taken to prevent some of the common threats to valid findings. These include attributing undue importance to first impressions or dramatic events, such as focusing on a "juicy" quote, selectivity in choosing data to present, especially when trying to confirm key findings, and confusing correlation with causation.[7,8] Demonstrating that all text was reviewed and that multiple reviewers participated is a way of providing assurance to readers that data analysis was designed to avoid threats to validity.

In general, it is a good idea to have someone else read through the description of procedures to be sure that this section is clear and that steps have not been omitted. One should minimize the use of jargon and define terms that have a specific meaning for qualitative research. Terms such as "theme," "code," and "tag," among others, should always be defined. Qualitative researchers should assume that their reader may not be familiar with qualitative research methods. By explaining procedures so that non-qualitative readers will understand them, the author will increase the chance that the reader will understand and appreciate the substantial time and rigorous attention to detail that qualitative research requires. It is a common misconception among researchers unfamiliar with qualitative research, perhaps because it generally involves no equipment more sophisticated than a tape recorder, that qualitative research lacks analytical rigor.[9] Careful descriptions of methods in qualitative research manuscripts will help dispel this idea.

Presenting Findings

The data presentation is the heart of any paper, and qualitative researchers have many options for conveying their results. Whatever format is chosen, this section of the paper has only two purposes: to tell the reader what the researcher found out, and to communicate how the researcher knew that he or she was correct in the conclusions drawn. The author should choose a style that fits the particular study purpose and methods. One can present themes that emerge from the large body of data collected. Alternatively, one can focus on case studies that encapsulate complex ideas. It is important to provide enough detail to make the work real and alive. Achieving this goal is a challenge while keeping within the page or word constraints of a journal. It is also necessary to choose a technique for preserving each informant's anonymity. While the general outlines of this strategy are usually contained in the documents approved by the IRB, they need to be fully operationalized and described in the written paper. Often choosing a pseudonym is not enough to ensure informants' anonymity; one should decide whether and how revealing details needed to be changed for the published work.

The presentation of results often, but not always, involves the use of direct quotations from informants. Direct quotations can serve several functions, including the presentation of data to serve as evidence for conclusions and for conveying information about the speaker through the use of particular words and grammatical constructions. Quotations can be incorporated into the paper in different ways. Sometimes multiple short quotes are listed to provide evidence to justify a statement made by the researcher. These are often distinguished from the author's words by indenting. Sometimes informants' words or phrases are imbedded in the author's text and indicated with quotation marks. This use of the informants' words helps to support the author's point. Sometimes a single longer quotation is used, indented from the author's words. Such a quotation is used to convey complex ideas. Although an effective way of presenting data, these longer quotations often require a fair amount of the author's words to introduce and explain. Thus they are difficult to use except in a long paper. Whatever quotation style is chosen, a good strategy is to review the completed paper and be sure that each quotation is essential to making the point. If it is not, it can be eliminated.

Discussion and Conclusions

The final section of the paper should discuss the findings by summing up what has been learned. An effective paper discussion relates the findings to the background literature presented earlier in the paper and stresses what has been contributed that is new. Avoid claiming that the study is the "first" of anything. Be sure to comment on the study's limitations, whether in sample size, in method, or in the population to which it can be generalized. This is often a good transition to suggest where research should go next.

The Review Process

Most reviewer critiques highlight areas of the manuscript that might be unclear to a naïve reader or that need further development. It is not unusual to receive a review for a qualitative manuscript that indicates some or all of the reviewers are unfamiliar with methods and standards of qualitative research. Like all responses to reviewers, the response of a qualitative researcher should be polite and address the issues raised by each reviewer. One can assume that if the reviewer did not understand the paper, some readers of the journal will not either. Many non-qualitative researchers who review such papers are willing to learn more about qualitative research, and the author's response can help to educate the reviewer. The letter to the editor, describing the revisions made to the manuscript in response to the reviewers' comments, is a good place to put additional explanation that will not fit in the paper. For example, if the author says the way she or he has described the analysis is customary in qualitative research, providing citations of other examples in the peer-reviewed literature may be helpful to the reviewer. If a reviewer asks where the power analysis is, an author can describe the process for determining that the number of respondents is adequate and for reaching conclusions in qualitative research. The author should remember that it is not unreasonable for a reviewer to want to be assured that the analysis was as objective as possible.

Some reviewers' criticisms for a qualitative paper may be the result of another qualitative researcher faulting an author for taking one qualitative approach (e.g., phenomenology) rather than another (e.g., grounded theory). Because an editor without background in qualitative research is likely not to know the difference and therefore have to assume the reviewer is correct, the author needs to include a rationale for his or her approach in the response to the editor.

It is sometimes tempting to simply make changes suggested by reviewers who do not understand qualitative research. This might include counting up responses in focus groups to put a quantitative veneer on the work. While this is easy to do, it is usually scientifically not justified and may undermine the quality of the work. Taking the time to explain the fallacy of such data presentation to a reviewer (e.g., that a talkative focus group participant will be over-represented and a shy one under-represented) is a better solution. Another area that reviewers sometimes criticize is direct quotations that include slang or bad grammar, as the reviewer feels that it degrades the informant. The qualitative author should carefully review the material and consider how to convey respect for the informant without misquoting. However, editing quotations to make them more palatable is no more justified than a quantitative researcher changing numbers in a table to remove outliers. The quotations are the data on which findings are based and cannot simply be changed to suit the author or reviewer's taste.

Many papers are initially rejected by the first journal to which they are submitted. This happens to all authors, whether they are reporting on qualitative or quantitative research. Authors should consider the comments in the reviews from the rejecting journal and make changes to the paper to improve it before sending the manuscript to a second journal. This strategy is particularly important in qualitative research because the pool of reviewers is sometimes quite small for a particular topic area, such as gerontology. The small size of the reviewer pool means the paper may be reviewed again by the same reviewer(s) when submitted to another journal. If a reviewer encounters a paper substantially unchanged despite constructive critique provided in the original review, he or she is not likely to look kindly on the paper the second time.

Final Thoughts

Qualitative research is an important component of the overall research enterprise in social gerontology and in public health. Publication of findings can sometimes be challenging because much of the scientific literature and traditions in publishing are oriented to quantitative research. While this will undoubtedly change as more scholars do research, today's qualitative researchers need to expend extra effort to get their work into print. It is reassuring to note that as qualitative research has become more widely known, and as more qualitative research is published in "mainstream" journals, editors, reviewers, and readers are becoming more sophisticated consumers.

Although this chapter has given some tips on preparing a qualitative manuscript for publication, it is good to remember that qualitative manuscripts do not have to be written from a single formula, as is sometimes the case for quantitative studies. This distinction is both liberating and challenging. In the end, the best way to understand the construction of effective and compelling qualitative papers is to read them. Reviewing the literature regularly for good qualitative work and carefully examining how the papers were written is a worthwhile exercise for both students and professionals. Qualitative research has much to add to the knowledge base in gerontology and public health. Qualitative researchers can each be advocates for publication of these findings by writing and submitting manuscripts of high quality and on topics of keen interest.

Summary Points
- Publication of qualitative research findings can sometimes be challenging because much of the scientific literature and traditions in publishing are oriented to quantitative research.
- Challenges to publication of qualitative research include: 1) deviations from standard templates for structuring the manuscript may reduce the likelihood of acceptance, 2) researchers may not have a strong sense of how qualitative research should be written for publication, and 3) journal editors and reviewers may not be familiar with qualitative research.
- Minimum components for a manuscript include a problem statement, a conceptual framework, description of methods, a report of findings, and a discussion of what the findings mean.

References

1) Cheang, M. Older Adults' Frequent Visits to a Fast-Food Restaurant: Nonobligatory Social Interaction and the Significance of Play in a "Third Place." *Journal of Aging Studies.* 2002; 16:303-321.
2) Creswell, J.W. *Qualitative Inquiry and Research Design: Choosing among Five Traditions.* Thousand Oaks, CA: Sage Publications, 1998.
3) Quandt, S.A., et al. Meaning and Management of Food Security Among Rural Elders. *Journal of Applied Gerontology.* 2001; 20:356-376.
4) Quandt, S.A. and Rao, P. Hunger and Food Security Among Older Adults in a Rural Community. *Human Organization.* 1999; 58:28-35.
5) Mitteness, L.S. and Barker, J.C. Stigmatizing a "Normal" Condition: Urinary Incontinence in Late Life. *Medical Anthropology Quarterly.* 1995; 9:188-210.
6) Mitteness, L.A. So What Do You Expect When You're 85? Urinary Incontinence in Late Life. *Research in the Sociology of Health Care.* 1987; 6:177-219.
7) Krathwohl, G.R. *Methods of Educational and Social Science Research: An Integrated Approach.* White Plains, NY: Longman, 1993.
8) Miles, M., Huberman, A.M. *Qualitative Data Analysis. An Expanded Sourcebook.* Thousand Oaks, CA: Sage, 1994.
9) Gubrium JF. Qualitative Research Comes of Age in Gerontology. *Gerontologist.* 1992; 32: 581-582.

Acknowledgments This work was supported by grants from the National Institute on Aging (R01 AG13469, R01 AG17587). A shorter version of this paper was presented at a pre-conference workshop at the annual meeting of the Gerontological Society of America, "Qualitative and Mixed Methods Research: Improving the Quality of Science and Addressing Health Disparities." Washington, DC, November 19, 2004.

Chapter 13

A Publishable Manuscript:
One Editor's Experience and Recommendations

Linda S. Noelker, PhD

Introduction

The purpose of this chapter is to explain what can be done to increase the likelihood that qualitative and mixed-methods research manuscripts will be accepted and published in peer-reviewed scientific journals. To accomplish this, a review of research manuscript submissions to *The Gerontologist* was conducted to compare differences in the volume and disposition of manuscripts using quantitative methods with those using qualitative and mixed methods. The major reasons why qualitative research submissions were rejected also were examined. Results indicate that researchers using qualitative and mixed methods should clearly specify the purpose of the research and what it adds to the scientific literature, provide sufficient detail about the methodology, and explain the applied value of the research so readers are not left asking, "so what?"

A daunting challenge for a journal editor is being receptive to a far-ranging array of substantive topics and methodological approaches to scientific inquiry, while remaining true to the journal's mission and managing the realities of the publication process including page limits and backlogs. As soon as I became Editor-in-Chief of *The Gerontologist* in August 2002, inquiries started coming in as to whether or not I would publish articles based on qualitative research. These inquiries seemed peculiar at first because I couldn't conceive of a rationale for rejecting a particular methodological approach out of hand. However, after acquiring some months of editorial experience, it appeared that submissions based on qualitative research had a higher rejection rate than those based on quantitative research. The reasons for this differential disposition of manuscripts were unclear. Was this because of an unacknowledged bias against or ignorance of qualitative research on my part, or among the editorial board members who shoulder the bulk of responsibility for reviews? Or were there inadequacies in these submissions in terms of the quality of the research or explication of the methods in relation to the research purpose?

Research Manuscript Submissions

The following section provides a summary of review of the disposition of research manuscripts using quantitative, qualitative, and mixed methods that were submitted for consideration as research articles to *The Gerontologist*. (Submissions to Practice Concepts, Forum pieces or Brief Reports, and non-research manuscripts such as conceptual pieces are excluded from this analysis.) From August 1, 2002 through February 28, 2005, a total of 791 such manuscripts were received, and the overall number of submissions also has been increasing annually from a total of 282 in 2000 to over 400 in 2004. The largest increase to date was in 2004 when submissions jumped to 409 from 353 in 2003, with an additional 56 submissions.

Regarding capacity to publish, there are six issues of *The Gerontologist* published annually (excluding Special Issues). Each has between 144 and 156 pages with approximately 124 to 136 pages allocated for articles, resulting in about 75 to 80 articles published each year depending on the page lengths of the different articles in the volume. Obviously, with this capacity a relatively small portion of submitted manuscripts is published. In fact, the acceptance rate for quantitative manuscripts submitted from August 1, 2002 through February 28, 2005 was 17% compared to 12% for qualitative manuscripts submitted during this period, and this point will be elaborated further.

A comparison of the disposition of the 791 research manuscripts by type of method that were submitted for initial review by the Editor-in-Chief is shown in Table 1. The percentages of both types sent out by the editor for review are comparable (39% of the qualitative and 37% of the quantitative submissions), as are the percentages rejected without being sent for review.

Equal percentages of both types (16%) were sent back to the authors for revision before they went out for review. The reasons are myriad but a common one is that authors do not follow the format instructions for *The Gerontologist* that are published in each issue (e.g., exceeds word limit, does not follow APA guidelines). Additionally, manuscripts are returned if the practice and/or policy implications of the research are not addressed. As an applied aging research journal, articles published in *The Gerontologist* must have an applied focus with the research's implications for aging services, programs, clinical practice, and/or public policy clearly articulated at least in the discussion section, if not in the introductory section as well. Another reason is that the manuscript is not carefully edited (e.g., poorly written, typographical or grammatical errors) or filled with obscure acronyms that readers who are unfamiliar with the particular area of research will be challenged to keep in mind. Reviewers (and editors) become understandably frustrated if not offended by being asked to review poorly edited manuscripts, and authors are likely to shoot themselves in the foot by submitting unpolished work.

A comparison of the disposition of peer-reviewed manuscripts by type of method is shown in Table 2. About equal percentages of the qualitative and quantitative manuscripts are rejected after peer review (47% and 46%, respectively). A smaller percentage of qualitative compared to quantitative submissions were accepted for publication (22% and 34%, respectively), however, almost twice as large a percentage of qualitative submissions are currently in review (31% compared to 17%). The reason for this phenomenon is clear from the data in Table 3 showing that the number of qualitative

Table 1. Disposition of Submitted Research Manuscripts (N = 791) by Type of Method Used (8/1/02 through 2/28/05)

	Qualitative/Mixed Methods		Quantitative Methods	
	%	(n)	%	(n)
Sent for review when received	39	(34)	37	(260)
Rejected without review	45	(40)	47	(334)
Invited by editor to revise	16	(14)*	16	(109)
Total	100	(88)	100	(703)

*Of the qualitative manuscripts, 2 of the 14 were sent for review after initial revision and 68 of the 109 quantitative ones were sent. Thus, the total sent for review included 36 (41%) qualitative/mixed methods manuscripts and 328 (47%) of the quantitative manuscripts.

Table 2. Disposition of Peer-Reviewed Research Manuscripts (N = 364) by Type of Methods Used (8/1/02 through 2/28/05)

	Qualitative/Mixed Methods		Quantitative Methods	
	%	(n)	%	(n)
Accepted	22	(8)	34	(110)
Rejected after review	47	(17)	46	(151)
Currently in review/revision	31	(11)*	17	(56)
Withdrawn	0		3	(11)
Total	100	(36)	100	(328)

Table 3. Annual Number of Submitted Qualitative/Mixed-Methods Manuscripts

Year	Number	
2002	13	(8/1/02 through 12/31/02)
2003	26	
2004	42	
2005	42*	

*Projected based on 7 submissions in first two months of 2005.

submissions was quite low until 2004 when they increased to 42 from 26 in 2003. A sizable portion of these manuscripts remains either in revision or review, thus evidence about actual differences in acceptance rates by type of method is not yet available.

Reasons for Rejection

Qualitative or mixed-methods manuscripts are rejected for publication for several reasons: inadequate conceptual basis or justification for the study, incomplete or inappropriate methods, and interpretation of findings that reach beyond the data. Each of these reasons will be discussed in greater detail.

Inadequate justification. The primary reason for rejection of a qualitative or mixed-methods manuscript is that the conceptual basis for the research is not carefully explained nor its purpose clearly specified. This phenomenon is illustrated by the following comments (paraphrased) written by reviewers in their reports to authors. "No explanation is given for why this study is needed and what it adds to the literature." "The author's taxonomy is not moored to theory or conceptual schemes already in the literature."

Experts recommend authors pay thorough attention to specific aims, background, and significance in order to increase the odds of having qualitative research funded and published in scientific journals.[1,2] Although qualitative studies typically do not include hypotheses and tend to be broader in scope and more fluid in methods, authors need to place the research within the larger body of extant scientific literature, and this includes prior qualitative and quantitative investigations that are relevant. Unless the author displays a thorough knowledge of this literature and clearly identifies gaps, inconsistencies, or limitations that the research was designed to address, reviewers will not understand the contribution it makes to the scientific literature. Both qualitative and quantitative researchers should make certain that this section does not read like a literature review. The purpose is not to convince editors and reviewers that every related investigation has been read and understood; the referenced literature should be used to underscore the importance of the research, the conceptual approach used, and exactly what it adds to the literature. Lastly, editors are likely to be concerned when none of the literature cited in manuscripts was published in their journals.

Methodological limitations. An equally prominent reason for the rejection of qualitative and mixed-methods manuscripts is that the methods are inadequately explained or are unsound. The following comments (paraphrased) by reviewers illustrate these points: "The authors fail to embrace the major design feature: dyadic responses." "How many interviewers were there? How were they trained? Are there any concerns about interviewer bias?" "How many researchers did the analysis? Were external people involved in reviewing the analysis or the code structure? Was there an audit trail of analytic decisions?" "How were disconfirming cases handled?"

Incomplete or unclear reporting of methods is a frequent reason for rejection of qualitative submissions, which is disheartening because this section should highlight and clearly illustrate the unique contribution that qualitative methods make to gerontological knowledge. The section should present a compelling case for why only the specific procedures employed in the study could produce the desired knowledge. Hence, the methods have to tie back to the research's purpose and research questions. Simply to state that a "grounded theory" approach or a particular software program was used for analysis does not address the critical issues of why and how. As another example, a typical statement about data collection is that data were gathered until "saturation" was reached, but the decision criteria for saturation are unspecified. Lastly, it is not uncommon for qualitative researchers to ignore the limitations of their research, fail to report refusal rates, and not detail why procedures or design features were changed during the investigation (e.g., adding new research sites).

Overstated findings. The third reason why qualitative and mixed-methods submissions are rejected from publication in *The Gerontologist* is the findings and conclusions overreach the data and the applied value of the research is not explicated. The following comment by a reviewer illustrates this problem. "The implications for family therapy are rather narrow. It would be interesting if the authors could at least offer some ideas about the implications for future research as this is often a goal of exploratory studies." The reviewers and I should never be left asking "so what?" regarding exactly what the research adds to the literature or the rationale for submitting it to a particular journal.

The Substantive Focus of Qualitative Research Submissions

One of my concerns about the rejection of qualitative and mixed-methods submissions was that a pattern would be found in the rejection of manuscripts dealing with particular topics or certain older populations such as HIV/AIDS patients or substance and drug abusers. An examination of the substantive focus of the 88 qualitative submissions was conducted; however, a comparison of those that were rejected without review, rejected after review, and accepted was not possible because, as noted earlier, a large portion are currently in review and/or revision.

Of the 88 qualitative research articles submitted to *The Gerontologist* since August 2002, the most common focus was on issues in nursing homes and other congregate residential settings (over 30 submissions). Over half of these submissions concerned direct care workforce or family caregiver issues such as affective care work by nursing assistants, the perceived quality of family visits with residents, and family perspectives on end-of-life care. There were 13 submissions focused on how a diagnosis of dementia is communicated to patients and/or their family members and how decisions about care are made in advanced dementia or at end of life. Although many submissions could be cross-categorized because they addressed several topics, submissions related to dementia, caregiving, and residential care were most numerous. Surprisingly, only seven submissions concerned special populations such as gay, lesbian, bisexual, or transgendered older adults, those with HIV/AIDS, and the homeless when qualitative methods would appear to be well suited to research on these groups.

It should also be noted that 26 of the 88 qualitative and mixed-methods submissions were from researchers in other nations. Unfortunately, a considerable number of these manuscripts were awkwardly written because English was not the author's first language. Even when it was indicated in the manuscript that editorial assistance was obtained from a professional service, the expression of aging research concepts and methods is not easily translatable. Furthermore, this problem is not confined to qualitative and mixed-methods submissions but applies to quantitative research articles submitted by authors from non-English-speaking nations as well. This problem also is encountered by other editors of the Gerontological Society's journals, and there does not appear to be an easy solution.

Conclusions

This chapter characterized one editor's experience with qualitative and mixed-methods manuscript submissions in the hope that researchers will gain a better understanding of how to better prepare manuscripts for submission and thus increase their chances for publication in this forum. The limitations of qualitative manuscripts and recommendations for improving them described here are consistent with those offered by others for obtaining grants and publishing findings based on qualitative methods in scientific journals.[1-5] Clarity of purpose, specificity about where the study fits in the larger scientific literature, rationale for specific methods in relation to research purpose, clear and complete description of the methods, and reporting the limitations of the research are all essential components of a well-prepared manuscript.

There is an additional issue about qualitative and mixed-method research submissions for which there is no easy solution: longer length that typically exceeds the allowable word count for research articles (for example, 6,000 words in *The Gerontologist*). Several authors have made cogent arguments for having their manuscripts accepted even though they exceed the word limit, arguing the additional space is required in order to provide sufficient detail about the methods and other aspects of the research. However, the editorial staff must struggle with this issue because it affects the timing of page availability for authors whose articles were accepted and are waiting to see their work in print. For this reason, all authors, whether their research uses quantitative or qualitative methods, should be circumspect about the manuscript's length.

Lastly, this chapter on manuscript submissions, rejections, and acceptance for publication in *The Gerontologist* is intended to help new investigators in particular better understand the competition around publication in peer-reviewed journals. It takes substantial practice to learn how to prepare a manuscript for publication and good mentoring is essential. Thus it is a great pleasure to read a well-prepared manuscript that has a new investigator as lead author with well-established gerontologists trailing behind and, conversely, greatly disappointing when the manuscript is not well done.

Aside from preparing research manuscripts, another excellent way to acquire experience at publishing is to serve as a reviewer of these manuscripts. *The Gerontologist* is acquiring a cadre of "novice reviewers" (graduate and post-doctoral students and new investigators) who serve as a third or fourth reviewer of a manuscript and benefit from seeing the other reviewers' critiques in comparison with their own. Often, the lessons learned from others' mistakes can be as valuable as lessons learned from your own.

Summary Points
• Manuscripts based on qualitative research may have a higher rejection rate than those based on quantitative research due to unacknowledged biases of editors or reviewers or inadequacies in these submissions.
• Essential components of a well-prepared manuscript include clarity of purpose, specificity about where the study fits in the larger scientific literature, rationale for methods used, clear and complete description of the methods, and discussion of the study's limitations.
• Qualitative or mixed-methods manuscripts are rejected for publication for several reasons: inadequate conceptual basis or justification for the study, incomplete or inappropriate methods, and interpretation of findings not supported by the data.

References

1) Offices of Behavioral and Social Sciences Research, National Institutes of Health, Publication Number 02-5046, December 2001.
2) Belgrave, L., Zablotsky, D., and Guadagno, M. How do we Talk to Each Other? Writing Qualitative Research for Quantitative Readers. *Qualitative Health Research.* 2002; 12(10), 1427-1439.
3) Devers, K. How Will We Know "Good" Qualitative Research When We See It? *Health Services Research.* 1999; 24(5): 1153-1188.
4) Mays, N. and Pope, C. Assessing Quality in Qualitative Research. *British Medical Journal.* 2000; 320:50-52.
5) Patton, M. Enhancing the Quality and Credibility of Qualitative Analysis. *Health Services Research.* 1999; 34 (5): 1189-1208.

Acknowledgements I would like to express my sincere gratitude to Jeanne Hoban, Assistant Editor of *The Gerontologist*, for her assistance gathering the data for the tables, helpful comments and editing this manuscript, and her invaluable work processing the flow of submissions to *The Gerontologist*. Further, her unfailing good humor contributes enormously to the quality of my life as Editor-in-Chief and is much appreciated by authors, reviewers, and editorial board members.

Chapter 14

Informing Aging-Related Health Policy
Through Qualitative Research

Leslie A. Curry, PhD, MPH, Renée R. Shield, PhD, and Terrie Wetle, MS, PhD

Introduction

Despite increasing interest in evidence-based health policy, the impact of health and health services research on policy remains limited.[1-5] The translation of research findings into health policy has been constrained by a number of factors, including lack of timeliness or relevance of the research, differing incentives and priorities between academia and the public sector, lack of collaborative relationships among researchers and policymakers, and ineffective communication of study findings.[6,4] Within this broader context, qualitative investigations have traditionally been regarded with skepticism and are frequently viewed as the least useful form of research by policymakers.[7]

These challenges have been also observed with respect to aging-related research, where linkages among academia, government, and service providers are also tenuous.[8] However, scientifically sound qualitative research can not only play an important and unique role in state and federal aging-related health policy,[9,8] but the theoretical and methodological perspectives inherent in qualitative approaches provide essential data that cannot be gathered with quantitative methods. This chapter provides rationale for the importance of these methodologies and offers guidance for researchers interested in designing, conducting, and disseminating qualitative research to inform policy.

The chapter is organized into five sections. First, we briefly describe the potential contributions qualitative research can make to aging-related policy. Second, we discuss approaches to enhancing policymakers' confidence in evidence generated through qualitative methodologies. Third, we examine strategies for building essential relationships between the research and aging health policy communities. Fourth, we present communication techniques that can enhance the effectiveness of disseminating research findings to policymakers. Illustrative case studies or examples from the empirical literature are provided throughout the chapter.

Potential Contributions of Qualitative Research to Health Policy in Aging

The influence of any given study on state or national health policy is difficult to determine, although there is general consensus that immediate and explicit impact is the exception rather than the norm.[10] The link between research and policy may be characterized as direct, enlightening, or selective in nature.[11] *Direct* links result in specific and observable application of the research findings to a policy or program. As an example, the development of the Minimum Data Set (MDS) for nursing home residents was based on both quantitative and qualitative analyses which were used to develop and test the various MDS measures.[12,13,14] Reporting on MDS measures is now required by the Centers for Medicare and Medicaid Services, and the data are now used as part of quality assurance strategies as well as to provide information to the public regarding individual nursing facilities. Research plays an *enlightening* function when it generally enriches the understanding of an issue and implications of various policy decisions. An example of this enlightening function would be the continued research on the PACE (Program of All-inclusive Care of the Elderly) programs as they are implemented across the country (http://www.cms.hhs.gov/researchers/demos/PACE.asp). A *selective* relationship occurs in cases where data are used to give credibility to predetermined positions. An example of this is the development of the federally funded Older Americans Act congregate meals program. Although a demonstration project designed to evaluate the acceptability and effectiveness of meals programs for older persons had not yet been completed, the full program was funded by Congress and researchers were then asked to provide data regarding the effectiveness of the demonstration projects after the fact. While this sort of "selective" data application is clearly not a desired outcome from the researcher's perspective, both direct impact and enlightening relationships can make important contributions to the development and implementation of health policy.

Qualitative research can serve a unique and critical role, both in complementing quantitative approaches, as well as in addressing questions for which quantitative techniques are not appropriate. Examples of areas best explored through qualitative approaches include understanding individual values, preferences, and perspectives, particularly in vulnerable or marginalized populations; defining social norms and expectations; evaluating program or policy implementation; and characterizing processes of organizational change.[7,15]

The following examples from aging research illustrate the distinct nature of qualitative data. A study of family involvement in decisions with nursing home residents combed large-scale participant observation with quantitative analysis of interviews across four contrasting nursing facilities.[16] Findings demonstrated that families play a substantial and integral role in such decisions, in contrast to the widespread perception that families and their elderly members have superficial ties with one another. Using participant observation and qualitative interviews, Shield[17] has demonstrated how family members interact with staff members in several nursing homes, both to forge alliances with staff members and to advocate for their relative. One mixed-methods study of physical abuse of older adults used open, as well as close-ended, questions and a variety of scales to test several theories of elder abuse.

The qualitative data described the interpersonal relationships between abuser and abused, added to information that helps explain why victims stay with abusers, and expounded on data derived from quantitative sources alone.[18] Finally, qualitative interviews following a large national quantitative survey more fully characterized how family members experience the end-of-life care of their loved ones in nursing homes.[19]

Qualitative anthropological research has provided considerable evidence of the importance of many aging and health constructs often unexamined by policymakers. Standard conceptions of Alzheimer's and other dementing diseases are challenged by those who describe the cultural discourse in which cognitive deficits are framed and the variety of meanings the symptoms have to diverse populations.[20,21] The differences in how menopause is experienced by women throughout the world (see, for example, the chapter by Beyene in this volume) underscore the powerful and complex interaction of culture, biology, nutrition, and ecology. Such explorations into the connotations and experiences that aging and health have within different groups help us understand how health policy can be better tailored to diverse populations. The refinement in our understanding of illness, health behaviors, and experiences related to aging contributes to more appropriate and effective policy and health care interventions.

Furthermore, qualitative research can provide information that is particularly relevant for each stage of the policy cycle: formulation, implementation, and evaluation.[22] With early stages of policy formulation, a qualitative study might define the phenomenon or issue of interest, consider relevant policies and programs, and illuminate implications of various policy approaches. For example, when the Connecticut legislature was considering changes to state Medicaid policy regarding asset tests for nursing home eligibility, a study was commissioned to examine the magnitude and prevalence of intentional transfer of assets to qualify for Medicaid (known as "Medicaid estate planning").[23] Medicaid eligibility workers participated in a series of focus groups, which are well suited for exploring topics about which little is known, or which involve personal and social constructs.[24] Findings described factors influencing Medicaid estate planning, problems in enforcement of regulations, and recommendations for improved policy responses. One such recommendation, revision of formulas for determining "penalty periods," was subsequently incorporated into state policy.

At the implementation stage, qualitative methods are especially valuable in characterizing processes and assessing organizational and community responsiveness. For example, one qualitative study explored implementation of the Patient Self-Determination Act (PSDA) in nursing homes.[25] In-depth interviews were completed with a purposeful sample of health care professionals to elicit detailed descriptions of their experiences and perceptions regarding implementation of the law. A range of impediments to successful implementation were identified, including the institutional commitment to the PSDA, the breadth of advance care planning efforts, challenges to incorporating advance care planning into the admission process, difficulties in assessing residents' capacity to participate in discussions, issues regarding family compliance with residents' wishes, and limited staff knowledge regarding advance directives. The study was considered by the Connecticut Coalition to Improve End-of-Life Care in its deliberations regarding state policies for advance care planning.

Finally, evaluation of a policy or program may examine its impact on individuals, communities, or organizations, and document unanticipated outcomes. For example, the qualitative work by Shield et al.[19] assessed the impact of hospice care in nursing homes from the point of view of close family members. In-depth interviews with fifty-four close family members and friends of those who spent some time of the last month of life in a nursing home indicated the generally positive effect of hospice care in the nursing home, and generated revealing stories of how the terminal phases of life were experienced by the decedents and their families.

Synthesis of qualitative studies. In order to ensure access to the full range of published qualitative studies, improved methods for searching, identifying, and appraising such studies are needed. A number of frameworks for synthesis of qualitative data (also known as cross-case analysis) have been developed, including meta-ethnography[26] and meta-synthesis.[27] Meta-ethnography involves selecting relevant empirical studies, reading them repeatedly and noting down key concepts (or "interpretive metaphors"), which then are synthesized into overarching constructs. There is no consensus regarding the acceptability of synthesizing qualitative studies, as this strategy relies on an assumption of generalizibility that is not uniformly endorsed by qualitative researchers.[28]

Although qualitative research alone can certainly generate critical information, in some instances integration of quantitative and qualitative studies together may more appropriately characterize a multifaceted phenomenon. For example, policymakers seeking to understand barriers to access community-based, long-term care will need to draw on qualitative evidence characterizing individual perceptions of filial caregiving responsibilities, as well as quantitative evidence regarding service structure and financing. Systematic and rigorous methods for synthesizing qualitative and quantitative forms of evidence are essential, although little work has been done in this area.

The potential value of qualitative research to policy can be maximized through considered and deliberate efforts on three broad fronts. First, qualitative researchers must enhance policymakers' confidence in research findings by ensuring that studies are conceived and conducted in a scientifically sound manner and meet commonly accepted criteria for quality. Second, researchers (and their academic institutions) must invest in and sustain collaborative relationships with policymakers to ensure that research questions are relevant and that findings are appropriately included in policy formulation. Third, translation and communication of research findings must be timely and effective with diverse audiences of policymakers at various levels. The remainder of the chapter will address each of these strategies.

Enhancing Policymakers' Confidence in Qualitative Research

There is considerable debate among qualitative researchers as to whether standardized criteria for assessing the quality of qualitative studies are appropriate.[29] Over the past decade, guidelines for assessing the rigor of qualitative research have been developed across a range of scientific disciplines.[25,30,31] While there is great variability among these approaches, the following constructs are frequently addressed in some form: validity and reliability of the data (also referred to as trustworthiness and authenticity), and generalizability of the findings (or transferability).[25,32] There is also general consensus about the following broad quality criteria: explicitly stated aims/objectives of the research; appropriate use of qualitative methods; appropriate sample design for qualitative research and explicit selection criteria; clarity about the analytic process; and clarity about how the evidence and conclusions are derived.[33] In studies using participant observation, researchers are cautioned to be explicitly aware of boundaries between the researcher as observer and participant, to provide thorough documentation of observations and other data, to create an audit trail, and to verify comparisons among multiple observers and/or interviewers.[34] A comprehensive discussion of issues of research quality is beyond the scope of this chapter. For further consideration of validity and reliability in qualitative and mixed-method research, see chapters in this volume by Morgan and Morse.

Some argue that societal relevance of the research is as important as scientific rigor, and standards for assessing the salience of research to policy development have been proposed.[1] Major domains and associated potential indicators focus on the priority of the policy issue, translation of the issue into a feasible research question for which there are appropriate methods, degree of cooperation between researchers and policymakers, potential contribution of the findings, and likelihood of effective dissemination.

The utility of qualitative research in particular for policy may be assessed in accordance with a framework proposed by Spencer and colleagues.[33] In order for the research to be perceived as valuable by policymakers, it must: 1) contribute to a deeper understanding of a phenomenon; 2) employ a research strategy which can address the evaluation questions posed; 3) be systematic and transparent in collection, analysis and interpretation of qualitative data; and 4) offer well-founded and plausible arguments about the significance of the data generated. These four conditions are global enough to apply to most forms of qualitative investigation. Moreover, the authors define 18 appraisal questions and associated quality indicators that relate more specifically to focus groups, in-depth interviews, document analysis, and observation. Readers with particular interest in the area of criteria for policy relevance for qualitative research are encouraged to read the excellent, comprehensive report by Spencer and colleagues.[33]

Overarching guidelines for quality have been met with ambivalence by some experts, who caution that disproportionate emphasis on use of specific techniques (such as respondent validation or triangulation) may sacrifice a study's potential value (or, result in the "tail wagging the dog").[35] Nevertheless, many argue that it is essential for qualitative studies to meet some standards of quality in design, conduct, and reporting in order to allay policymakers' concerns that this type of research is not "scientific."[7,30,1]

Building Relationships Among Researchers and Policymakers

Impediments to the development of research-policy-practice partnerships are well documented.[36–8] Traditionally, researchers and policymakers have struggled with significant linguistic, cultural, and professional differences that pose challenges to the creation of mutual trust and respect.[8] Tensions have been described by the "two-communities thesis," which suggests that social scientists perceive themselves as rational and objective, and view decision-makers as interest-oriented and indifferent to evidence. Conversely, decision-makers consider themselves to be action-oriented and pragmatic, and view scientists as naïve and jargon-ridden.[39] Although most researchers feel their work has relevance to policymakers, most policymakers do not regard the research community as particularly helpful in policy development.[5] Researchers are trained to focus on the complexity of issues, to qualify their conclusions, to identify alternative interpretations of the data, and to acknowledge the limitations of their work. Such complexities and qualifications are often not well tolerated in the policy arena, although appreciation for these ambiguities is important for effective policy formulation.[5]

In addition to these individual perceptions and attitudes, institutional incentives and pressures differ in the two environments. Professional accomplishment in academe is primarily measured by publication in peer-reviewed journals, most of which impose an embargo on the release of findings until the article has appeared in print. Additionally, academic journals are not the optimal venue for reaching policymakers.[1] Researchers must adhere to institutional processes that are often lengthy, such as satisfying institutional review board requirements and complying with staffing policies for grant-supported activities, and that may impede their ability to conduct a study in time to inform policy. In contrast, service providers or policymakers have pragmatic and immediate needs, require timely information, and because of the need to make immediate decisions, may be required to rely on the "best available" evidence, regardless of whether it is definitive or conclusive.

Despite these obstacles, collaborative relationships that do manage to thrive may offer a number of mutual benefits. Sustained dialogue and interaction build rapport and facilitate the researcher becoming a trusted source. Successful partnerships require that investigators demonstrate an ongoing commitment to meaningfully engaging policymakers and making findings readily accessible. Policymakers may contribute unique perspectives regarding critical research needs and objectives, as well as participate in the conceptualization and implementation of the research. Such involvement increases the likelihood the research will be relevant, timely, and used to inform policy. Bringing these constituencies together also increases understanding of differing demands and incentives.[36,2] From an institutional perspective, formal relationships can provide a vehicle for payers, particularly Medicaid programs, to make data available to researchers, as well as offer opportunities to secure funding from a variety of sources.[40,8]

One example of a partnership among researchers, policymakers and providers in the field of aging is that between Institute for Health Policy, Edmund S. Muskie School of Public Service, University of Southern Maine, MaineCare, and the Maine Department of Human Services (access Institute for Health Policy at: http://muskie.usm.maine.edu/research/research_institutes_ihp.jsp). This successful consortium conducts a wide range of applied health and health services research projects that directly inform state policy. For example, the state of Maine had concerns regarding the continuity of care in nursing homes, as reflected by an observed pattern of frequent cycling of residents between nursing homes and the community. Based on a collaborative research effort that characterized the nature and magnitude of the problem, state policy was developed to facilitate continued nursing home residence for the target population at risk.[40] Another example is a collaboration between Brown University, the state of Rhode Island's office of the Attorney General and Department of Elderly Affairs, Blue Cross/Blue Shield, and several institutions across the state, to improve end-of-life care (http://www.chcr.brown.edu/dying/BROWNATLAS.HTM). Brown-based research documented many concerns regarding end-of-life care, including failure to execute or heed advance directives, problems in symptom management including pain control, and difficulties in achieving patient and family wishes in clinical decision-making. Researchers collaborated with policymakers from the Attorney General's office and the Department of Elderly Affairs to develop a document entitled "Choices and Conversations: A Guide to End-of-Life Care" that was published by the state's major newspaper, *The Providence Journal,* and delivered with the Sunday papers to most Rhode Island households.

While most collaborative arrangements among researchers, policymakers, and providers are formal contractual relationships, some are less structured in nature. For example, the Scripps Gerontology Center at Miami University of Ohio has contracts from both providers and policymakers, allowing it to serve a "broker" function. Brokers maintain relationships in both arenas and are therefore positioned to link policymakers with appropriate research centers or scientists with specific expertise (also referred to as "research brokers").[8] Scripps has long-standing relationships with the Knolls of Oxford, a continuing care community, and various state agencies in Ohio, including the Department of Aging.[40] Collaborative efforts rely on a variety of funding sources, including state governments, grants from foundations or the federal government, and endowments.

Several specific mechanisms have been recommended to facilitate successful linkages between the policy and research communities. Training of "policy entrepreneurs" (persons with seasoned research backgrounds who are familiar with university research organizations, but who also understand the policy process and can communicate effectively with state policymakers) has been encouraged.[36] Exchange programs or scholar-in-residence programs might be created to give researchers exposure to policy development and policymakers the opportunity to provide substantive input into research agendas.[41] Conferences, workshops, and other meetings that are carefully tailored to facilitate communication across the professional divide can be an effective and relatively efficient way to build researcher–policy-maker linkages.[8] Research institutions (particularly public universities) should provide incentives for faculty interested in bridging between academia and government.[1] Finally, funding agencies must become more amenable to supporting the translation of findings into dissemination formats more readily useable by policymakers.[41]

Effective Communication of Qualitative Research Findings

Even if the research is scientifically sound and credible, and a substantive, collaborative relationship exists between researchers and policymakers, a study cannot inform policymaking unless it is effectively communicated. While researchers are generally quite comfortable with presenting their empirical work in academic forums, very different skills are required to bring research into the policy process in such a manner as to achieve maximum impact.[36] Successful communication of research to policymakers requires thoughtful synthesis, translation, and dissemination of the essential aspect of the research findings.[8,42] Careful attention to the organization and content of information can facilitate use of findings. The following section of this chapter describes approaches to structure, content, and formatting of a research report intended for policymakers.

Structure

The research report must be organized to anticipate and meet the respective needs of different consumers within the policymaking environment. Known as "layering" of information, this format allows readers to access the scope and depth of information best suited to their needs. One useful approach has been developed by the Canadian Health Services Research Foundation (CHSRF, 2005), referred to as the 1:3:25 rule. According to this rule, a report should begin with one single page of bulleted "main messages," or lessons decision-makers can take from the research. The messages should not be simply a summary of empirical findings, but rather a clear and concise overview of the potential implications of findings. If the study's results are not conclusive, needs for future research should be defined. Next, a three-page executive summary should present the central findings of the study in concise, nontechnical language, with not more than a few sentences regarding methods and analysis. Finally, the complete report, which is most likely to be read by legislative staff responsible for more in-depth understanding of the evidence, should be approximately 25 pages in length.

Language and Content

A guiding principle for content in research-based policy reports is clarity. Study aims and objectives, the analytical process, and the construction of evidence and conclusions must each be presented with great precision and clarity.[33] The substance of the report should be communicated in a direct manner, with minimal jargon. Social science has been aptly referred to as a "terminological jungle,"[43] and the field of qualitative research methods suffers from lack of a unifying language to an even greater degree.[33] A term such as "grounded theory" is a case in point. Its very different meanings range from an inclusive definition including any qualitative study that uses inductive techniques, to a much narrower definition that follows Glaser and Strauss's work[44] and views any deviation as "not grounded theory."[45] It is acceptable to use appropriate technical terms, but they should be defined for the reader. While technical terms used appropriately and judiciously increase clarity and precision, their proliferation can lead to confusion instead.

The report should address the following content. The study's context should be briefly laid out, stating the research objective clearly and explaining how this study adds to the existing literature. The salience of the research to current policy deliberations must be explicitly stated and readily apparent to the reader. Methods must be reported with sufficient detail to be credible, but without exhaustive attention to minutiae that might be provided in an appendix or companion document available upon request. The summary of major results should reflect main themes and may also include graphic or tabular information. Tables and figures must be clear and informatively titled; quotations, headings, and underlining may also be used to emphasize critical points.[42,46] Limitations of the study should be enumerated, including potential barriers to translating the research into practice. Policymakers understand the challenges inherent in conducting research and will accept limitations of studies when the limitations are presented clearly.[46] Policymakers also indicate that they expect to see policy implications from the researcher's perspective, but are not interested in speculation that reaches far beyond the data.[8] Needs for future research should be articulated that identify gaps in knowledge and suggest studies to address those gaps. Finally, other supportive material may be included in appendices, such as related resources (publications, websites and other useful sources of information).

The following example illustrates the importance of timely research that is directly responsive to policymakers' expressed needs. Amidst controversy over the feasibility of expanding a pilot program of personal care assistants for residents over 65, the Connecticut Department of Social Services (DSS) commissioned a study to evaluate the pilot.[47] The study, completed in four months, included in-depth interviews with key informants who represented all stakeholders, program clients, and individuals who chose not to enroll. Preliminary cost impact estimates were also calculated. The final report began with an executive summary that clearly defined the purpose of the study, identified collaborators (which included DSS staff), and gave an overview of the study's primary components. The executive summary highlighted the findings of greatest interest to DSS, the perceptions of program participants regarding program benefits, and recommendations for improvements. Although the findings were preliminary, the summary reported the cost-effectiveness data since the legislature was extremely interested in this information. The full report was fifty-nine pages long; appendices included data collection instruments for the key informant, participant and family interviews, as well as references and selected resources. The report informed the deliberations of the state's Long Term Care Planning Committee, and the pilot program has since been expanded.

Conclusion

Qualitative research represents an underutilized resource for informing the implementation of innovative and practical policy initiatives. There are a number of approaches qualitative researchers might employ to facilitate the greater application of their work in these areas. First, it is essential to ensure that policymakers perceive the research as timely, relevant, and of high quality. Done well, qualitative research offers unique and important opportunities to inform the policy formulation, implementation, and evaluation. Second, it is becoming clear that substantive collaborations with policymakers, while time-intensive and not generally valued in academe, are critical to the design and conduct of timely and relevant research. Finally, the communication of research findings must be tailored to the interests and needs of policymakers and reported in an appropriate way via an accessible format. As interest in qualitative research continues to grow, consideration of the strategies described in this chapter are likely to enhance its value for and application to aging-related policy. The need for clear and effective aging policy cannot be over-estimated, and qualitative methods provide powerful tools for providing relevant and necessary information to policymakers.

Summary Points
- Current contributions of qualitative and mixed-methods research to policy are limited by a number of factors, including lack of timeliness or relevance of the research, differing incentives and priorities between academia and the public sector, lack of collaborative relationships among researchers and policymakers, and ineffective communication of study findings.
- Qualitative and mixed-methods research can provide important and unique information to policymakers at each stage of policy development: formulation, implementation, and evaluation.
- Qualitative researchers must enhance policymakers' confidence in research findings by ensuring that studies are conceived and conducted in a scientifically sound manner.
- Researchers (and their academic institutions) must invest in and sustain collaborative relationships with policymakers.
- Translation and communication of research findings must be timely and effective with diverse audiences of policymakers.

References

1) Bensing, J.M. et al. Doing the Right Thing and Doing it Right: Toward a Framework for Assessing the Policy Relevance of Health Services Research. *International Journal of Technology Assessment and Health Care.* 2003;19(4):604-12.

2) Davis, P. and Howden-Chapman, P. Translating Research Findings into Health Policy. *Social Science and Medicine.* 1996;43(5):865-72.

3) Harries, U., Elliott, H., and Higgins, A. Evidence-Based Policymaking in the NHS: Exploring the Interface Between Research and the Commissioning Process. *Journal of Public Health Medicine.* 1999;21:29–36.

4) Lohr, K., Eleazer, K., and Mauskopf, J. Health Policy Issues and Applications for Evidence-Based Medicine and Clinical Practice Guidelines. *Health Policy.* 1998; 46:1-19.

5) Roos, N.P. and Shapiro, N. From Research to Policy: What Have We Learned? *Medical Care.* 1999; 37:JS 291-305.

6) Innvaer, S., Vist, G., Trommald, M., and Oxman, A. Health Policy-Makers' Perceptions of Their Use of Evidence: A Systematic Review. *Journal of Health Services Research and Policy.* 2002;7(4):239-44.

7) Leys, M. Health Care Policy: Qualitative Evidence and Health Technology Assessment. *Health Policy.* 2003; 65: 217-226.

8) Feldman, P., Nadash, P., and Gursen, M. Improving Communication Between Researchers and Policy Makers in Long Term Care, or Researchers are from Mars, Policy Makers are from Venus. *The Gerontologist.* 2001; 41(3):312-321.

9) Almarsdottir, A.B. and Traulsen, J.M. Studying and Evaluating Pharmaceutical Policy—Becoming a Part of the Policy and Consultative Process. *Pharm World Sci.* 2006, Jun 30; [online publication]

10) Lavis, J., Ross, S., and Hurley, J. Examining the Role of Health Services Research in Public Policymaking. *Milbank Quarterly.* 2002; 80(1):125-154.

11) Elliott, H. and Popay, J. How are Policymakers Using Evidence? Models of Research Utilization and Local NHS Policymaking. *Journal of Epidemiology and Community Health.* 2000; 54:461-468.

12) Morris, J.N., Hawes, C., Fries, B.E., et al. Designing the National Resident Assessment Instrument for Nursing Homes. *The Gerontologist.* 1990;30:293-307.

13) Hawes, K. et al., Reliability Estimates for the Minimum Data Set for Nursing Home Residents Assessment and Care Screening. *The Gerontologist.* 1995; 35:172-178.

14) Mor, V. et al. Inter-Rater Reliability of Nursing Home Quality Indicators in the U.S. BMC. *Health Services Research.* 2003;3(1):20.

15) Sofaer, S. Qualitative Methods: What are They and Why Use Them? *Health Services Research.* 1999;34:1101-8.

16) Rowles, G.D. and High, D.M. Family Involvement in Nursing Homes: A Decision-Making Perspective. In: Stafford, P., (Ed.) *Gray Areas: Ethnographic Encounters with Nursing Home Culture.* Santa Fe: SAR Press; 2003: 173-201.

17) Shield, R.R. Wary Partners: Family-CNA Relationships in Nursing Homes. In: Stafford, P. (Ed.) *Gray Areas: Ethnographic Encounters with Nursing Home Culture.* Santa Fe: SAR Press; 2003: 203-233.

18) Pillemer, K. Combining Qualitative and Quantitative Data in the Study of Elder Abuse. In Reinharz, S. and Rowles, G.D. (Eds.) *Qualitative Gerontology.* 1988; New York: Springer.

19) Shield, R. et al. 2005. Physicians "Missing in Action:" Family Perspectives on Physician and Staffing Problems in End-of-Life Care in the Nursing Home. *Journal of the American Geriatrics Society* 53 (10): 1651-1657.

20) Gubrium, J. and Sankar, A., (Eds.) *Qualitative Methods in Aging Research.* Thousand Oaks: Sage; 1994.

21) Cohen, L. *No Aging in India: Alzheimer's, the Bad Family, and Other Modern Things.* Berkeley, CA: University of California Press; 1998.

22) Rist, R.C. Influencing the Policy Process with Qualitative Research. In Denzin, N. and Lincoln, Y. (Eds.) *Handbook of Qualitative Research.* Thousand Oaks, CA: Sage Publications, Inc. 1994: 545-557.

23) Walker, L., Gruman, C., and Robison, J. Medicaid Eligibility Workers Discuss Medicaid Estate Planning for Nursing Home Care. *The Gerontologist.* 1999; 39(2):201-208.

24) Kruger, R.A. and Casey, M.A. *Focus Groups: A Practical Guide for Applied Research* (3rd ed). Thousand Oaks, CA: Sage; 2000.

25) Walker, L., Bradley, E., Blechner, B., and Wetle, T. Problems in Implementing the Patient Self-Determination Act in Nursing Homes. *Journal of Mental Health and Aging.* 1998; 4(1):83-96.

26) Noblit, G.W. and Hare, R.D. Meta-Ethnography: Synthesizing Qualitative Studies. London: Sage Publications; 1988.

27) Sandelowski, M., Docherty, S., and Emden, C. Qualitative Metasynthesis: Issues and Techniques. *Research in Nursing and Health.* 1997; 20, 365–371.

28) Campbell, R., Pound, P., Pope, C. et al. Evaluating Meta-Ethnography: A Synthesis of Qualitative Research on Lay Experiences of Diabetes and Diabetes Care. *Social Science & Medicine.* 2003; 56:671–684

29) Mays, N. and Pope, C. Assessing Quality in Qualitative Research. *British Medical Journal.* 2000; 320:50-52.

30) Popay, J., Rogers, A., and Williams, G. Rationale and Standards for the Systematic Review of Qualitative Literature in Health Services Research. *Qualitative Health Research.* 1998; 8(3):341-351.

31) Devers, K. How Will We Know Good Qualitative Research When We See It? *Health Services Research.* 1999; 25(5):1153-1188.

32) Patton, M. Enhancing the Quality and Credibility of Qualitative Analysis. *Health Services Research.* 1999; 34(5):1189-1208.

33) Spencer, L., Ritchie, J., Lewis, J., and Dillon, L. Quality in Qualitative Evaluation: A Framework for Assessing Qualitative Research. 2003 Available at: http://www.policyhub.gov.uk/evalpolicy/qual_eval.asp.

34) Ulin, P.R., Robinson, E.T., and Tolley, E.E. *Qualitative Methods in Public Health: A Field Guide for Applied Research.* San Francisco: Jossey-Bass: 2005.

35) Barbour, R.S. Checklists for Improving Rigour in Qualitative Research: A Case of the Tail Wagging the Dog. *British Medical Journal.* 2001; 322, 1115–1117.

36) Coburn, A. The Role of Health Services Research in Developing State Health Policy. *Health Affairs.* 1998; 17(1):139-151.

37) Ross, S. et al. Partnership Experiences: Involving Decision-Makers in the Research Process. *Journal of Health Services Research and Policy.* 2003; 8 Suppl 2:26-34.

38) Shulock, N. The Paradox of Policy Analysis: If It Is Not Used, Why Do We Produce So Much Of It? *Journal of Policy Analysis and Management.* 1999; 18, 226–244.

39) Caplan, N., Morrison, A., and Stambaugh, R.J. *The Use of Social Science Knowledge in Policy Decisions at the National Level: A Report to Respondents.* Ann Arbor, MI: The University of Michigan, 1975.

40) Rogal, D. and McDaniel, L. *Long Term Care: Collaborating for Solutions.* Issue Brief. AcademyHealth: Washington, DC; 2003.

41) Feldman, P. and Kane, R. Strengthening Research to Improve the Practice and Management of Long Term Care. *Milbank Quarterly.* 2003; 81(2):179-220.

42) Dill, A. Writing for the Right Audience. In Gubrium J & Sankar A (Eds.) *Qualitative Methods in Aging Research*. Thousand Oaks, CA: Sage Publishers, 1994: 227-240.

43) Lofland, J., Lofland, L.H. *Analyzing Social Settings: A Guide to Qualitative Observation and Analysis* (3rd ed.). Belmont, CA: Wadsworth; 1995.

44) Glaser, B. and Strauss, A. *The Discovery of Grounded Theory: Strategies for Qualitative Research*. Chicago: Aldine; 1967.

45) Belgrave, L., Zablotsky, D., and Guadagno, M. How Do We Talk To Each Other? Writing Qualitative Research For Quantitative Readers. *Qualitative Health Research*. 2002; 12(10): 1427-1439.

46) Sorian, R. and Baugh, T. Power of Information: Closing the Gap Between Research and Policy. When it Comes to Conveying Complex Information to Busy Policy-Makers, a Picture is Truly Worth a Thousand Words. *Health Affairs*. 2002; 21(2):264-73.

47) Curry, L., Gruman, C., Porter, M., and Fogel, D. *Personal Care Assistant Pilot: Program Evaluation*. Developed for Connecticut Department of Social Services. 2001. Available at: http://www.hcbs.org/files/7/338/PCA_report_final.pdf. Accessed Sept. 19, 2005.

Index

Agency for Health Research and Quality (AHRQ), 142
Aging. *See* Gerontology
Aging-related health policy, informing through qualitative research, 183–195
Alzheimer's disease, theorizing method of research, 20–21
Analysis approach, choice of software, 119
Anthropology
  Autoethnography, 22–23
  comparative analysis, 105
  contribution to health studies, 103–106
  participant observation, 15–17, 105
  qualitative research of aging and health, 185
  role of the interviewer, 104–105
  social networks, 79–87
Archival data, qualitative public health study, 109–111
ATLAS.ti, 118–129, 126*f*, 129–134
  Code Output Report, *133*, 133–134
  combination of codes, 135–136
  diagramming ideas, 136–137, 137*f*
  memo writing, 127–128, 128*f*
  personalized workspace, ATLAS.ti, 129*f*
  screen view, 129–130

Bengtson and Morgan Los Angeles study, 82
Biological and cultural factors, 108

Canadian Health Services Research Foundation (CHSRF), 190
Center for Scientific Review (CSR), NIH grant proposals, 156
Coding transcripts
  Code books, 130–133, 131*f*
  Code combinations, 135–136
  Code exploration, 137–138
  Code review, *133*, 133–134
  Code types, 94–95, 94*t*
  Code weights, 132, 132*f*
  development, 92–95

double coding, 95
  initial scheme, 92–93
  linking codes to theory, 95–99
  revising and finalizing, 93
  types of codes, 94–95, 94*t*
Codework, 128–129
Coding schemes and data
  developing conceptual models, 98–99
Cognitive interviews, 40–41, 43
Combining qualitative and quantitative methods, *See also* Gerontology, Mixed Method Research, 64–65, 53–63
Comparative methods, in reproductive aging study, 106–108
Comprehensive Assessment and Referral Evaluation (CARE) survey, 86–87
Computer Retrieval of Information on Scientific Projects (CRISP), 146
Conceptualization and design, 6–7
  connected contributions, 53–63
  validity for mixed-method design, 65–77
Conceptual models, 98–99, 99*f*
  using qualitative methods, 4
Core component, in mixed-method design, 66–67
Cross-cultural comparisons, 106–108
Cultural diversity, qualitative research, 28
Cultural integrity, preserving through analysis, 103–115
Data analysis
  codes to theory, 91–102
  principles of and steps in, 91–92
  in reproductive aging study, 106–108
  sort and sift: think and shift, 122–124, 123*f*
Demographics, filtering by, 134
Department of Health and Human Services (DHHS), 142-143
Design criteria, 32–33
Diagramming ideas, 136-137, 137*f*

Ecological data, qualitative public health study, 109–111

Episode profiles, shaping of, 138
Ethnic/racial diversity, *See also*
    Anthropology
    autoethnography, 22–23
    cultural integrity, 103–115
    NIH grants and, 141–164
ETHNOGRAPH, 119–124
    combination of codes, 135–136
Ethnometric approach, 84–87
    establishing cultural relevance, 85
Evidence-based practice, using qualitative methods, 2–3
Expanded coverage, combining methods, 64

Filtering, by demographics, 134
Focus groups, 45–46

Gerontologist, The, 175–181
    reasons for rejection, 177–179
    research manuscript submissions, 175–177, 177*t*
    substantive focus of submissions, 179–180
Gerontology
    comparative methods and data analysis, 106–108
    multidisciplinary movement, 80
    qualitative data collection methods, 39–52, 80
    relevance of qualitative research, 16
    synchronizing qualitative and quantitative research, 79–89
    use of social networks, aging, and well-being to study, 80–83
Grant applications, NIH, 149–150

Health policy, potential contributions of qualitative research, 183–186
Highlighting text, MAXqda, 124, 125*f*
HyperQual, 119–121
HyperResearch, 119–121

In-depth interviews, 15–17
Inspiration and Decision Explorer, 119–121
Interviewer, role in qualitative research, 104–105
Interviews, 39–44
    cognitive, 40

key informant, 39–40, 43
number of participants, 42–44
qualitative public health study, 109–111
semi-structured/questionnaires, 74
structure, 40–41
unstructured, non-standardized, 73
variation in collection of data, 40

Journals. *See also* Manuscript preparation
    preparing a publishable manuscript, 165–168
    review process, 172–173

Manuscript preparation, 165–174, 175–181
    describing procedures, 169–171
    discussion and conclusions, 172
    journal choice, 165–168, 175–181
    presenting findings, 171
    reasons for rejection, 177–179
    review process, 172–173
    stating the problem and purpose, 168
    substantive focus of submissions, 179–180
MAXqda, 119–125, 125*f*, 129–134
    combination of codes, 135–136, 136*f*
    retrieved segments, 134, 134*f*
Memo writing, ATLAS.ti and MAXqda, 127–128, 128*f*
Minimum Data Set (MDS), nursing home residents, 184
Mixed method research, 53–63, 65–77
    advancing, 27–37
    connected contributions, 54–55
    maintaining validity, 68–72
    multi-method design, 67
    nomenclature for design, 66
    principles and procedures of validity for design, 65–78
    role of the supplementary strategy, 68–69, 69*f*
    substantive focus of submissions to journals, 179–180
    triangulation, 53–54
Mock review, NIH grant applications, 155–156
Mode of administration, qualitative interviews, 44

National Cancer Institute (NCI), 142
National Heart, Lung, and Blood
    Institute (NHLBI), 142
National Institute for Nursing Research
    (NINR), 142, 145
National Institute of Aging (NIA), 142,
    144–145
National Institute of Mental Health
    (NIMH), 142
National Institutes of Health (NIH)
    distinctions among grant mecha-
        nisms, 148*t*, 149
    funding of qualitative research at,
        146–147, 147*t*
    grant applications, 149–150
    institutes and centers at, 144*t*
    mock review of grant applications,
        155–156
    peer review process, 156–159
    PHS 398 Form, 149–155
    processing grant proposals, 156
    qualitative research at, 141–144
    RFAs and PAs, 149
    targeting an institute for a grant pro-
        posal, 145–146, 146*t*
    writing credible and fundable pro-
        posals, 141–164
National Science Foundation (NSF), 142
Network Analysis Profile (NAP), 85–86
NVIVO, 119–121

Observation
    as a data collection method, 47–48
    participant observation, 15–17, 105
Older Americans Act, 184

PACE (Program of All-inclusive Care of
    the Elderly) programs, 184
Participant observation, 15–17, 105
Patient Self-Determination Act (PSDA),
    185
Peer review, at NIH, 156–159
Policymakers
    confidence in qualitative research,
        187–188
    relationships with researchers,
        188–189
Primary method, methodological
    assumptions of, 70–71
Probes, in interviews, 41

Program Announcements (PAs), NIH, 149
Proposal writing, 141–164
Public Health Service (PHS) 398 Form,
    149–150
    research plan sections, 150–155
    tips for preparation, 163–164

Qualitative data, 39–52
    collecting for QUAL+quan, 73–74
    collecting separately, 76–77
    decisions, 48–50
    range of methods, 39–48
Qualitative research methods
    building conceptual models, 4
    codes to theory, 91–102
    credibility and vigor of, 29
    cultural context for, 27–29, 27–37
    effective communication, 8
    effective communication of findings,
        190–192
    funding at NIH, 146–147, 147*t*
    historical context, 16
    informing aging-related health poli-
        cy, 183–195
    integrating software, 117–139
    need for improved quality and cred-
        ibility, 5–6
    NIH, 141–144
    potential contributions to health pol-
        icy in aging, 183–186
    racially and ethnic diverse popula-
        tions, 1–2
    relevance for gerontology, 17
    synchronizing with quantitative
        research, 79–89
    theorizing method, 17–21
    enhancing QUAL description, 72–73
    threats to validity, 72
Quantitative research methods
    synchronizing with qualitative
        research, 79–89
    synthesizing with qualitative meth-
        ods, 4–5
    using qualitative research for devel-
        opment, 3–4
Question sequences, in interviews, 41

Rehabilitation, research projects, 28
Reproducibility and generalizability, in
    qualitative methods, 5

Request for Applications (RFAs), NIH,
    149
Researcher bias, in qualitative methods,
    5
Research Interviewing, Mishler, Elliot, 19

Scientifically sound analysis, planning
    and implementing, 7–8
Scientific Review Group (SRG), NIH
    grant proposals, 156
Scripts, in focus groups, 45–46
Self-awareness, researcher, 15–17
Sequence, 55*f*
Social and Cultural Contexts on Aging
    study, 81–82
Social disparity, qualitative research, 28
Social networks
    aging and well-being, 80–83
    depiction of, 21–22
    ethnometric approach, 84–87
    linkage attributes, 86
    member attributes, 86
    structure attributes, 86
    survey approaches to, 81–83
Software
    analysis approach to choice of, 119
    ATLAS.ti, 118–129, 126*f,* 129–134

choice of, 118–122
Codework, 128–129
ETHNOGRAPH, 119–124
    HyperQual, 119–121
MAXqda, 119–125, 125*f,* 129–134,
    135–136, 136*f*
NVIVO, 119–121
integrating with qualitative analysis,
    117–139

Sort and shift cycle, 122–124, 123*f*
State of the art, definition, 118, 122
Supplementary component, in mixed-
    method design, 66–67

Taxonomies, for linking code to theory,
    96–97, 97*f*
Textual and visual material analysis,
    increased reflexivity, 15–17
Triangulation, combining methods,
    53–54

Vogel's Qualitative Inorganic Analysis, 30

List of Contributors

Yewoubdar Beyene, PhD
Institute for Health and Aging
University of California San Francisco

Elizabeth H. Bradley, PhD
Department of Epidemiology and Public Health
Yale University

Katherine Bussinger, BA
College of Nursing
The University of Iowa

Leslie A. Curry PhD, MPH
Department of Medicine
University of Connecticut School of Medicine

Nancy Goldsmith, BA
College of Nursing
The University of Iowa

Jaber F. Gubrium, PhD
Department of Sociology
University of Missouri-Columbia

Mark Luborsky, PhD
Institute of Gerontology
Wayne State University

Stacie Salsbury Lyons, MSN, RN
College of Nursing
The University of Iowa

Raymond C. Maietta, PhD
ResearchTalk Inc.
Bohemia, NY

David L. Morgan, PhD
College of Liberal Arts and Sciences
Portland State University

Janice M. Morse, PhD (Nurse), PhD (Anthro), D (Nurse)
International Institute for Qualitative Methodology
University of Alberta

Linda Niehaus, PhD
International Institute for Qualitative Methodology
University of Alberta

Linda S. Noelker, PhD
Benjamin Rose Institute and
Editor, The Gerontologist

Sara A. Quandt, PhD
Department of Epidemiology and Prevention
Wake Forest University School of Medicine

Andrea Sankar, PhD
Anthropology Department
Wayne State University

Renée Rose Shield, PhD
Center for Gerontology and Health Care Research
Brown University

Shoshanna Sofaer, DrPH
School of Public Affairs
Baruch College of City University of New York

Jay Sokolovsky, PhD
Department of Anthropology
University of Southern Florida

Toni Tripp-Reimer, PhD
College of Nursing
The University of Iowa

Terrie Wetle, MS, PhD
Program in Public Health
Brown University

Ruth R. Wolfe, MPH
International Institute for Qualitative Methodology
University of Alberta